Galveston Diet

Cookbook for Beginners

Quick and Easy Delicious Mouthwatering Anti-Inflammatory and Hormone Balancing Recipes for a Healthy Lifestyle

Lauren Nielsen

Warning-Disclaimer

The purpose of this book is to educate and entertain. The author or publisher does not guarantee that anyone following the techniques, suggestions, tips, ideas, or strategies will become successful. The author and publisher shall have either liability or responsibility to anyone with respect to any loss or damage caused, or alleged to be caused, directly or indirectly by the information contained in this book.

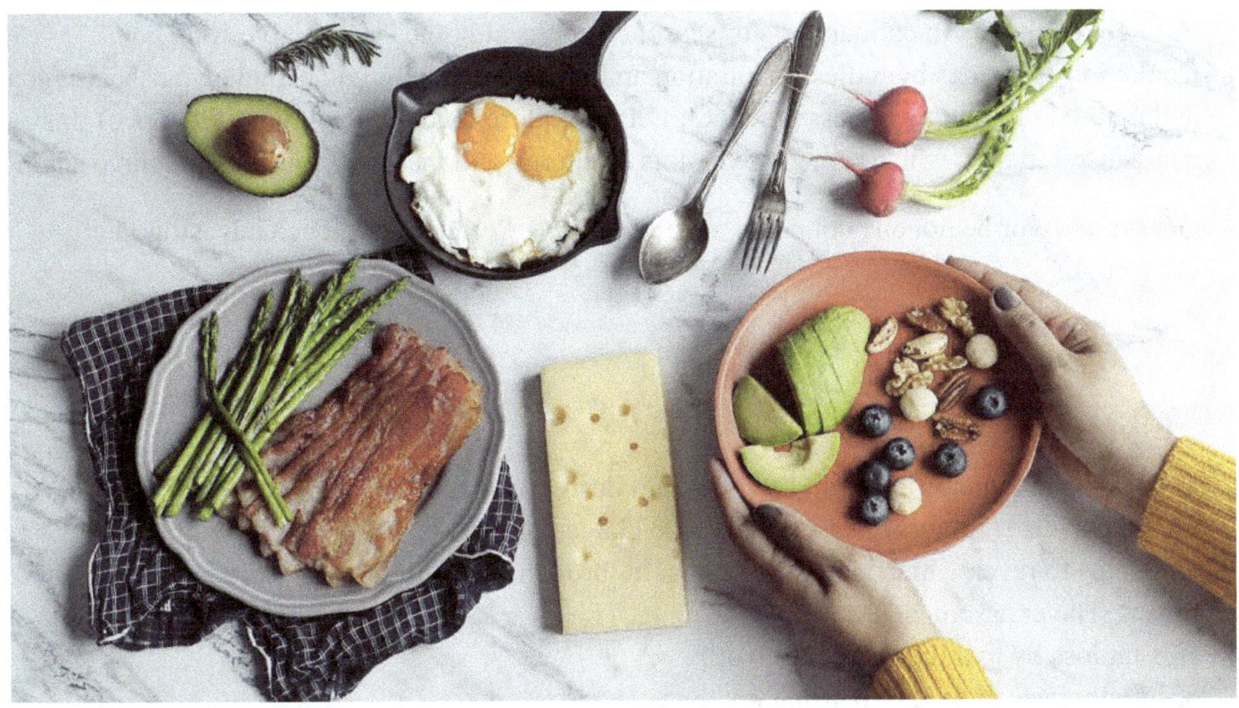

INTRODUCTION

Welcome to The Galveston Diet Cookbook,' the perfect gastronomic masterpiece designed to empower you using a transformative approach to healthy living. In this book, you are invited to take a tasty voyage that will promote vibrant well-being and make you enjoy cooking and eating delicious food.

The Galveston Diet, initially created by Dr. Mary Claire Haver, is much more than just a diet; it's a holistic lifestyle approach that has changed many people's lives for better health. Based on science and influenced by the beautiful coastal town of Galveston, Texas, this eating plan incorporates balanced meals, hormone optimization, and mindful eating.

This cookbook has a wealth of recipes that do not go well with the fundamental philosophy of the Galveston Diet. Traditionally referred to as our culinary experts, we have them carefully preparing various dishes so that they can satisfy your taste buds while at the same time nourishing your body from the inside. From hearty soups and bright salads to mouth-watering main courses and incredible sweets, each recipe was created with thought to maximize taste but not compromise nutrition.

However, this cookbook is more than just compiled recipes but rather a guide towards healthier and happier selves. The author gives us valuable information through every page on how to choose ingredients, plan our meals, and identify our serving sizes so that we can make sound decisions about our healthy future. We have also included Dr. Haver's insights explaining how each dish promotes total wellness based on the scientific principles behind the Galveston diet.

For both beginners in culinary arts or seasoned cooks at home, "The Galveston Diet Cookbook" provides boundless inspiration and guidance to help you achieve your health goals and maintain lifelong wellness practices. Let us explore together the unique flavors of this coast-inspired diet, which will give you lots of energy and make you vibrant and alive again.

Get set to savor health one delicious recipe at a time. Welcome to "The Galveston Diet Cookbook."

What is the Galveston Diet?

The Galveston Diet is a weight loss program designed specifically for women in the perimenopause and menopause stages. The Galveston Diet is a self-paced weight loss program that helps to reverse menopausal weight gain through anti-inflammatory foods and intermittent fasting. Haver asserts that this approach aids fat loss by making hormones work positively instead of just focusing on restricting calories. It emphasizes whole foods while limiting processed foods, added sugars, and artificial ingredients.

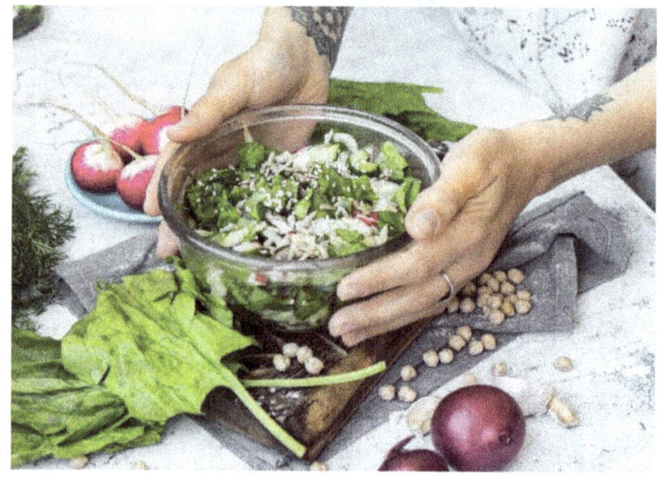

According to it, the diet should consist of whole foods that are not processed and contain abundant antioxidants and nutrients that reduce inflammation in the human body. This is believed to help counter hormonal imbalances and stubborn weight gain often experienced during menopause. Lean proteins, fruits, vegetables, legumes, whole grains, healthy fats, and full-fat dairy products come to mind first. Avoid processed foods, added sugars, artificial ingredients, and inflammatory oils.

This program uses a 16/8 intermittent fasting method where 8 hours are given for daily intake consumption, as all the remaining 16 hours are spent fasting. This strategy is thought to enhance metabolism so that fat, especially belly fat many women experience during menopause, is burned more efficiently.

Thus, the key thing about The Galveston Diet is changing your eating habits to feed your body correctly during the day. This includes prioritizing high-quality protein, healthy fats for satiety and energy, and moderate carbohydrates for a constant energy supply level. A reason why sugar as well as refined carbs are minimized is because they can cause blood sugar peaks leading to inflammation.

Health Benefits of the Galveston Diet

The Galveston Diet is a program intended for middle-aged women to help them lose weight and be healthy. Here are some of the essential health benefits:

Weight Loss and Fat Reduction:

Intermittent fasting results in reduced calorie intake, leading to metabolism optimization. This also helps in losing weight. Focusing on whole foods rich in nutrients and balanced macros increases satiety and prevents overeating, contributing to long-term weight management. The other advantage is that it reduces belly fat, a common problem during menopause.

Improved Hormonal Balance and Menopausal Symptoms:

Chronic inflammation is responsible for the imbalances in hormones due to menopause. On the other hand, this diet's anti-inflammatory nature may also help with hormone regulation that could lead to hot flashes, sleep disruption, and mood swings, among others. Balanced protein and healthy fats will support hormonal health while contributing to hormonal balance.

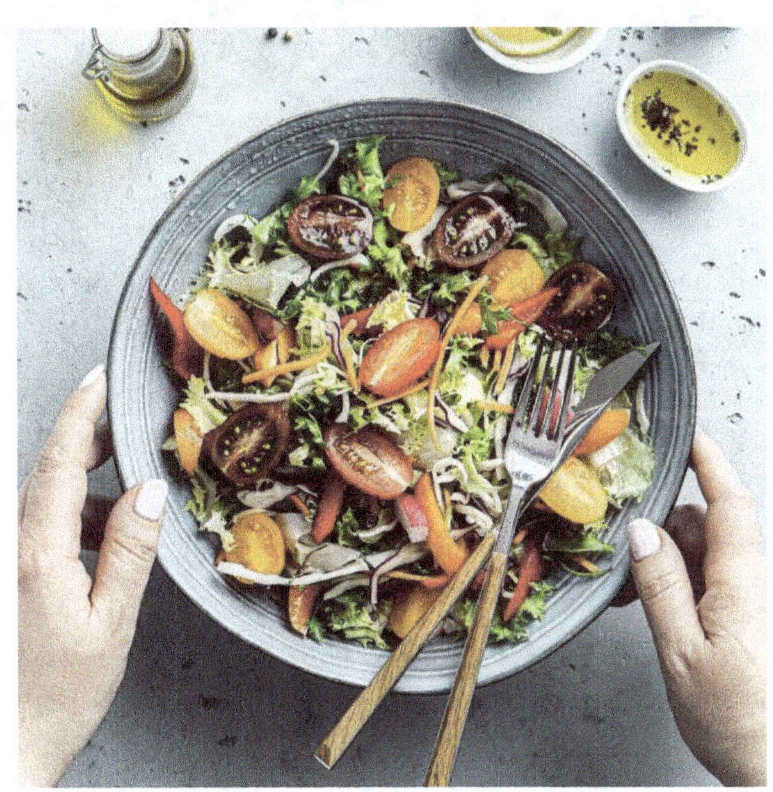

Reduced Inflammation and Chronic Disease Risk:

Inflammatory foods full of antioxidants counterbalance chronic inflammation, thus reducing the risk of numerous chronic diseases related to menopause, like heart disease, diabetes, and some cancers. Intermittent fasting can also reduce inflammation risk, lowering chronic conditions' chances.

Increased Energy Levels and Overall Well-being:

During sugar reduction, your blood sugar levels will stabilize so that you can enjoy constant energy all day. Sustained energy is found through healthy fats plus proteins and an overall focus on nutrient-rich foods that maintain optimal body functioning, leading to increased energy and, thus, better well-being overall.

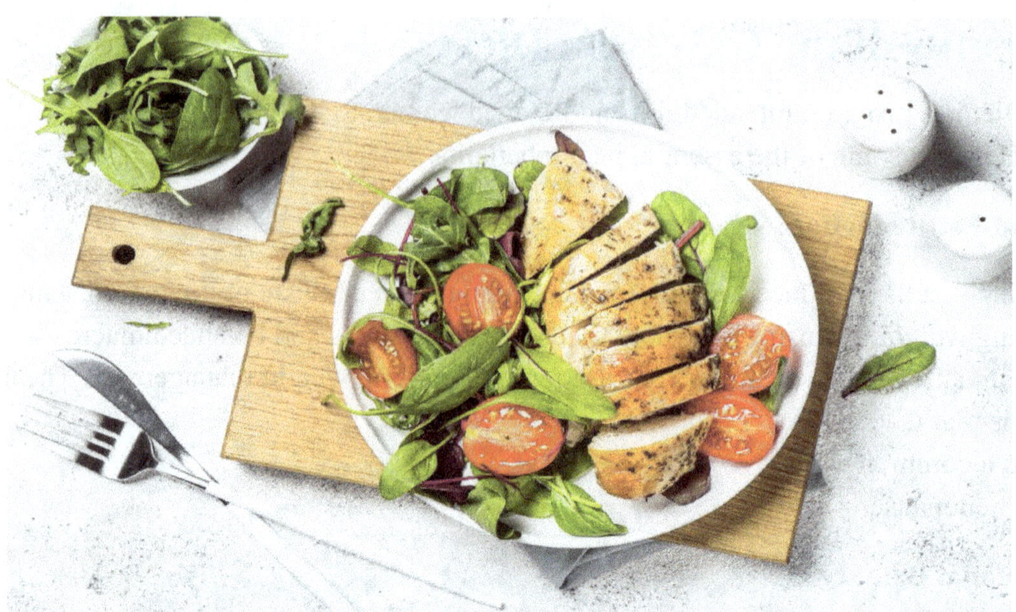

Food is allowed to be eaten on the Galveston Diet.

Whole and nutrient-dense foods are the focal point of the Galveston Diet, which emphasizes anti-inflammatory and hormone-balancing properties. The foods that are usually encouraged in this diet include the following:

Lean Proteins: Fish, poultry, eggs, and plant-based sources like beans and legumes are included. They help in muscle maintenance and general health.

Healthy Fats: These include avocados, olive oil, nuts and seeds. These fats are advantageous to the heart and may decrease inflammation.

Low-Glycemic Fruits and Vegetables: They have many vitamins, minerals, and fiber. This kind of fruit helps to moderate sugar levels in the blood.

Whole Grains: Preferably quinoa, brown rice, barley, etc., instead of refined grains, which provide necessary nutrients for maintaining a healthy digestive system.

Anti-Inflammatory Foods: Turmeric, ginger, berries, plus leafy greens, which have anti-inflammatory properties, are highly recommended.

Fermented Foods: It includes yogurt, kefir as well as sauerkraut, among others, that are good for your guts.

Hydration: Water intake is incredibly stressed for general health purposes and aiding weight loss.

Moderate Dairy: Small amounts of low-fat and fermented dairy products can be consumed.

Herbs and Spices: When used in meals, they do not supply extra calories or sodium.

Foods are not allowed on the Galveston Diet.

It is advised that you stay away from pro-inflammatory foods with no nutritional value because they can lead to weight gain while causing minimal benefits to your health. You may have heard about some of these already.

Processed Foods: They contain unhealthy fats, a lot of sodium, and preservatives, which can cause inflammation and contribute to weight gain.

Added Sugars: These comprise sugary beverages and high-sugar foods like candies, cakes, and cookies, among others. This leads to weight gain, spikes in blood sugar levels, and increased inflammation.

Refined Carbohydrates: Examples are white bread, white flour pasta, white rice, and other refined grains. They can be harmful due to their tendency to create a deviation in blood sugar levels that lacks nutrients.

High-Glycemic Fruits and Vegetables: Because of their propensity for spiking blood sugar levels, some fruits (potato) and vegetables (watermelon) with higher glycemic indices might be restricted.

Certain Fats and Oils: For example, the use of transfats and certain saturated fats found in fried foods, processed snacks, or baked goods should be limited since they are pro-inflammatory.

Alcohol: However, small amounts of particular types of alcohol, such as red wine, might be permissible; large quantities are not recommended.

High-Dairy Foods: Some versions of this diet may exclude high-fat dairy products as these can cause inflammation in some people who eat them.

Highly Caffeinated Beverages: In certain instances, though not always, too much caffeine consumption may be curtailed.

Certain Condiments and Sauces: Generally, condiments or sauces with lots of sugar, salt, or unhealthy fat content are avoided.

CHAPTER 1: BREAKFAST RECIPES

Egg White Waffles

Prep time: 5 minutes Cook time: 5-7 minutes Servings: 2

Ingredients

- 4 large egg whites
- 1/2 cup of unsweetened almond milk
- 1/4 cup of unsweetened applesauce
- 1/4 tsp vanilla extract
- 1/4 cup of oat flour
- 1/4 cup of almond flour
- 1/2 tsp baking powder
- 1/4 tsp cinnamon
- Pinch of salt

Optional toppings:

- Fresh berries (blueberries, raspberries, strawberries)
- Chopped nuts (almonds, walnuts, pecans)
- Nut butter (almond butter, peanut butter)
- Greek yogurt
- Sugar-free maple syrup (use sparingly)

Instructions

1. Preheat the waffle iron.
2. Whisk egg whites, almond milk, applesauce, and vanilla extract in a large bowl until frothy.
3. Whisk together oat flour, almond flour (or whole-wheat flour), baking powder, cinnamon and salt in another bowl.
4. Fold the dry ingredients gently into the wet ingredients just until mixed. Avoid over-mixing.
5. Spray the waffle iron with cooking spray if necessary
6. Pour batter onto the waffle iron and cook according to the instructions on your waffle iron.
7. Remove the waffles from the iron; warm them with your favorite toppings.

Nutrition:

Calories: 180 Fat: 5g Carbs: 20g Protein: 15g

Kale Scramble

Prep Time: 5 minutes Cook Time: 10 minutes Servings: 1

Ingredients

- 2 large eggs
- 1/4 cup of chopped kale (fresh or frozen)
- 1/4 cup of chopped onion
- 1/4 cup of chopped bell pepper (any color)
- 1/4 cup of chopped mushrooms
- 1 tbsp olive oil
- Salt and pepper to taste

- Kale Scramble

Instructions

1. Kale, onion, bell pepper, and mushrooms must be washed and chopped.
2. Heat olive oil in a non-stick pan over medium heat for sautéing. Then, add the onion and bell pepper; cook them for around 5 minutes until they soften.
3. Cook kale and mushrooms for 2-3 more minutes until kale wilts.
4. Beat the eggs together with salt and pepper in a bowl.
5. Pour vegetables into the egg mixture in the pan. Use a spatula to stir gently as you would wish your eggs to be cooked through.
6. The favorite toppings should be used when serving this kale scramble immediately.

Nutrition per serving

Calories: 200 Fat: 10g Carbs: 5g Protein: 15g

Veggie Omelet

Prep time: 5 minutes Cook time: 10 minutes Servings: 1

Ingredients

- 2 large eggs
- 1/4 cup of chopped bell pepper (any color)
- 1/4 cup of chopped onion
- 1/4 cup of chopped mushrooms
- 1/4 cup of chopped spinach
- 1 tbsp olive oil
- Salt and pepper to taste
- Optional toppings: crumbled feta cheese, avocado slices, salsa
- Veggie Omelet

Instructions

1. The bell pepper, onion, mushroom, and spinach should be washed and chopped.
2. Heat olive oil in a non-stick pan over medium heat. Add the onion and bell pepper, cooking for about 5 minutes until they become tender.
3. Add mushrooms and spinach, and cook for 2-3 minutes until the spinach is wilted.
4. In a bowl, whisk eggs, salt and pepper together.
5. Pour the egg mixture into the vegetables in the pan. Tilt the pan to spread out the egg mixture evenly.
6. Cook the omelet until set on the bottom (2-3 minutes). Using a spatula, gently fold the omelet in half.
7. Serve immediately with preferred toppings.

Nutrition per serving

Calories: 250 Fat: 12g Carbs: 5g Protein: 20g

Eggs with Spinach

Prep time: 5 minutes Cook time: 5 minutes
Serving: 1

Ingredients

- 2 large eggs
- 1/4 cup of chopped fresh spinach
- 1 tbsp olive oil
- Salt and pepper to taste

Instructions

1. In a bowl, beat eggs with salt and pepper.
2. Heat olive oil in a pan over medium heat.
3. Add spinach and cook until it wilts, about a minute or two.
4. Once you have done this, add the egg mixture and scramble it to your satisfaction.
5. Serve immediately.

Nutrition

Calories: 250, Fat: 15g, Carbs: 2g, Protein: 18g

Mushroom & Arugula Frittata

Prep time: 10 minutes Cook time: 25 minutes Servings: 4

Ingredients

- 4 large eggs
- 1/4 cup of unsweetened almond milk (or milk of choice)
- 1/4 tsp dried thyme
- Salt and pepper to taste
- 1 tbsp olive oil
- 1/2 cup of chopped onion
- 1/2 lb. sliced mushrooms
- 2 garlic cloves, minced
- 1/4 cup of chopped fresh arugula
- 2 oz. Crumbled goat cheese

Instructions

1. Preheat oven to 400°F (200°C).
2. Take a bowl, and in it, mix eggs and almond milk, thyme, salt, and pepper.
3. Place olive oil in a non-stick skillet that can also be used in the oven, then heat it over medium heat.
4. Add onions to the oil, then cook for about five minutes until they turn soft.
5. Brown mushrooms and garlic for 5-7 minutes or until tender.
6. At this point, add arugula and cook till wilted, but never overcook it.
7. Tilt the pan to spread the egg mixture evenly before pouring it inside. Then sprinkle goat cheese on top of it.
8. This skillet is later placed into an oven where it will bake for 15-20 minutes or until the top turns golden brown like an egg omelet and sets the egg entirely through.
9. Afterward, let it cool down slightly before you serve.

Nutrition per serving

Calories: 250 Fat: 15g Carbs: 5g Protein:

Blueberry Muffins

Prep time: 15 minutes Cook time: 18-20 minutes Servings: 12

Ingredients

- 1 1/2 cups of whole wheat flour
- 1/2 cup of almond flour (or oat flour)
- 1 tsp baking powder
- 1/4 tsp baking soda
- 1/4 tsp salt
- 1/4 cup of unsweetened applesauce
- 1/4 cup of coconut oil, melted
- 1/4 cup of honey
- 1 large egg
- 1 tsp vanilla extract
- 1 cup of fresh blueberries (or frozen)

Optional toppings

- Chopped nuts (pecans, walnuts, almonds)
- Sliced fresh fruit (bananas, strawberries)
- Sugar-free maple syrup

Instructions

1. Preheat oven to 375°F (190°C). Grease or line a muffin tin with 12 cups of.
2. Considering the dry ingredients include whole wheat flour, almond flour, baking powder, baking soda, and salt, whisk them together in a large bowl.
3. Mix applesauce, melted coconut oil, honey, egg, and vanilla extract in another bowl.
4. When adding the wet to the dry ingredients, stir until a soft lump is formed; don't over-mix.
5. Finally, you can gently fold in blueberries into the batter.
6. The cup should be filled with batter three-quarters of the way up.
7. After oven baking for about 18-20 minutes or when a toothpick comes out clean after inserting it in the center of a muffin, it may be removed from the oven.
8. Allow muffins to cool in a pan for a few minutes before transferring them to a wire rack for complete cooling.

Nutrition per muffin:

Calories: 180 Fat: 8g Carbs: 25g Protein: 5g

Chicken & Bell Pepper Muffins

Prep time: 15 minutes Cook time: 18-20 minutes Servings: 12

Ingredients

- 1 cup of cooked and shredded chicken breast (grilled, baked, or poached)
- 1/2 cup of chopped red bell pepper
- 1/2 cup of chopped green bell pepper
- 1/4 cup of chopped onion
- 1/2 cup of chopped zucchini (optional, adds moisture)
- 1/2 cup of whole wheat flour

- 1/4 cup of almond flour (or oat flour)
- 1/4 tsp baking powder
- 1/4 tsp baking soda
- 1/4 tsp salt
- 1/4 tsp black pepper
- 1/4 cup of unsweetened almond milk (or milk of choice)
- 1 large egg
- 1 tbsp olive oil

Optional additions

- 1/4 cup of chopped fresh herbs (parsley, basil, oregano)
- 1/4 cup of crumbled feta cheese
- Chopped nuts (pecans, walnuts, almonds)

Instructions

1. Preheat oven to 375°F (190°C). Grease or line a muffin tin with 12 cups of.
2. Chicken, bell peppers, onion, and zucchini (optional) are mixed in a large bowl.
3. Mix whole wheat flour, almond flour, baking powder, baking soda, salt, and pepper in another bowl.
4. Almond milk, egg, and olive oil should be whisked together in a small bowl.
5. Wet ingredients are added to dry ingredients and stirred just until mixed. Avoid overtaxing the mixture.
6. Gently stir in the chicken and vegetables.
7. Fill muffin cups approximately 3/4 of the way full with batter.
8. Sprinkle with optional toppings like herbs, cheese, or nuts if desired.
9. Bake for 18-20 minutes until a toothpick inserted in the center comes clean.
10. Allow muffins to cool in the pan briefly before transferring to wire racks to cool completely.

Nutrition per muffin

Calories: 150 Fat: 5g Carbs: 15g Protein: 12g

Spinach and Mushroom Omelette

Prep time: 5 minutes Cook time: 10 minutes Servings: 1

Ingredients

- 2 large eggs
- 1/4 cup of chopped fresh spinach
- 1/4 cup of sliced mushrooms
- 1/4 cup of chopped onion (optional)
- 1 tbsp olive oil
- Salt and pepper to taste
- Optional toppings: crumbled feta cheese, avocado slices, salsa

Instructions

1. Add spinach, mushrooms, and onions (optional) to wash and chop in a bowl.
2. Heat olive oil in a non-stick pan over medium heat. Put the onions (if applicable) to become tender for about three minutes.

3. Brown mushrooms until they are cooked; it will take approximately five minutes.
4. Spinach is added, then cooked until just wilted for only one minute.
5. Mix eggs, salt, and pepper in a separate bowl by whisking.
6. Pour the mixed eggs into the vegetables in the pan. Tilt the pan so that the egg mixture can spread evenly.
7. The omelet cooks for 2-3 minutes until the bottom sets. Use a spatula to gently fold the omelet in half.
8. Top your favorite ingredients on the spinach mushroom omelet, then serve immediately.

Nutrition per serving

Calories: 250 Fat: 12g Carbs: 5g
Protein: 20g

Quinoa Breakfast Bowl with Berries

Prep time: 5 minutes Cook time: 15-20 minutes Servings: 1

Ingredients

- 1/2 cup of rinsed quinoa
- 1 cup of unsweetened almond milk
- 1/4 cup of chopped mixed berries
- 1 tbsp chopped nuts
- 1/2 tsp ground cinnamon
- Pinch of salt
- **Optional toppings:** chia seeds, hemp seeds, chopped banana, drizzle of honey

Instructions

1. Place quinoa, almond milk, cinnamon, and salt in a small saucepan. Bring to a boil, then reduce heat, cover, and simmer for 15-20 minutes – until quinoa is cooked and fluffy.
2. Wash and chop the berries. (Additional flavor and crunch can be achieved by lightly toasting the nuts).
3. Divide the cooked quinoa among bowls. Add any desired toppings, such as berries or nuts.

Nutrition per serving

Calories: 250 Fat: 5g Carbs: 40g
Protein: 8g

Overnight Chia Seeds with Almond Milk

Prep time: 5 minutes Cook time: Overnight (at least 4 hours) Servings: 1

Ingredients

- 2 tbsp chia seeds
- 1 cup of unsweetened almond milk (or milk of choice)
- 1/4 tsp vanilla extract (optional)
- Pinch of cinnamon (optional)
- 1/4 cup of chopped fresh berries or sliced fruit of your choice (optional)
- 1 tbsp chopped nuts or seeds (optional)

Instructions

1. Mix the chia seeds, almond milk, vanilla extract (if desired), and cinnamon (if desired) in a jar or container that can be closed with a lid. Stir everything together well.
2. Put the lid on top of the jar and let it sit in the refrigerator for at least four hours or overnight for the best texture of chia pudding.
3. In the morning, stir up the chia pudding. If you like, add your favorite fruits, nuts, or seeds on top.
4. Cold overnight chia pudding is what delights you.

Nutrition per serving

Calories: 200 Fat: 5g Carbs: 10g
Protein: 4g

Avocado and Poached Egg Toast

Prep time: 5 minutes Cook time: 5 minutes Servings: 1

Ingredients

- 2 slices whole wheat bread
- 1/2 ripe avocado
- 1 large egg
- 2 tbsp white vinegar
- 1/4 tsp chili flakes (optional)
- Salt and pepper to taste
- Optional toppings: chopped fresh herbs (cilantro, parsley), crumbled feta cheese, hot sauce

Instructions

1. Toasting the bread adds a great texture and taste, so you can toast it in that steamer, oven, or broiler until golden brown.
2. Slice or mash avocado, then spread it on the toast.
3. Fill a saucepan with water and bring to a simmer. Add vinegar. Crack the egg into a small bowl, then gently slip it into the simmering water. Cook for 3-4 minutes until the whites are set but the yolk is still runny. Alternatively, use a special poaching device for a more foolproof method.
4. Gently place the poached egg on top of the avocado toast. Season with chili flakes (if desired), salt and pepper.
5. You can then garnish with your favorite toppings (if desired) and serve immediately.

Nutrition per serving

Calories: 350 Fat: 20g Carbs: 30g
Protein: 15g

Veggie Breakfast Hash

Prep time: 5 minutes Cook time: 10-12 minutes Servings: 1-2

Ingredients

- 1 tbsp olive oil
- 1/2 cup of chopped onion
- 1/2 cup of chopped bell pepper (any color)
- 1/2 cup of chopped mushrooms
- 1/2 cup of chopped zucchini (optional)
- 1/2 cup of chopped spinach
- 2 large eggs
- 1/4 tsp turmeric
- 1/4 tsp paprika
- Salt and pepper to taste
- *Optional toppings:* crumbled feta cheese, avocado slices, salsa

Instructions

1. Chop and wash onion, zucchini (if using), bell pepper, and mushrooms.
2. Heat olive oil in a non-stick skillet over medium heat, then add the onion and cook for about 5 minutes.
3. Add bell pepper and mushrooms and cook for another 5 minutes until it becomes soft.
4. Finally, fry it for another 2-3 minutes if you use zucchini.
5. Wilt spinach by cooking and adding spices like turmeric, paprika, salt, and pepper.
6. Two hollows should be created on the vegetable mixture.
7. Break an egg into each of these hollows.
8. Simmer with a lid on for 2-3 minutes or until the yolks are cooked to your desired doneness and the whites are set.
9. Transfer this veggie breakfast hash to plates and use your favorite toppings.

Nutrition per serving

Calories: 300 Fat: 12g Carbs: 20g Protein: 20g

Mixed Berries Protein Smoothie

Prep time: 5 minutes Cook time: None Servings: 1

Ingredients

- 1 cup of frozen mixed berries
- 1 cup of unsweetened almond milk
- 1 scoop plant-based protein powder
- 1/2 cup of spinach
- 1/4 cup of chopped avocado
- 1/2 tsp ground flaxseed
- 1/4 cup of ice cubes
- Pinch of cinnamon

Instructions

1. Blend all ingredients together in a blender until smooth and creamy.
2. If the mixture is too thick, add more almond milk or a little water. Otherwise, if it is runny, add extra ice cubes or some frozen fruit.
3. Well, we hope that you find this mixed berries protein smoothie delightful!

Nutrition per serving

Calories: 250 Fat: 10g Carbs: 25g
Protein: 20g

Almond Butter Banana Smoothie

Prep time: 5 minutes Cook time: None
Servings: 1

Ingredients

- 1 ripe banana, peeled and frozen
- 1/2 cup of unsweetened almond milk (or milk of choice)
- 2 tbsp almond butter
- 1/4 cup of chopped fresh spinach
- 1 tbsp chia seeds
- 1/4 tsp vanilla extract (optional)
- Pinch of cinnamon (optional)
- Ice cubes (optional)

Instructions

1. To make almond butter banana smoothie recipe, put all the ingredients in a blender and blend until smooth and creamy.
2. If the smoothie is too thick, add more almond milk or water. Add additional ice cubes or a frozen banana if it's too thin.
3. You will love your almond butter banana fresh!

Nutrition per serving

Calories: 250 Fat: 15g Carbs: 25g
Protein: 12g

Beet & Berries Smoothie Bowl

Prep time: 10 minutes Cook time: 5
minutes Servings: 1

Ingredients

Smoothie Base:

- 1/2 cup of cooked beetroot, chopped (canned or roasted)
- 1 cup of frozen mixed berries
- 1/2 cup of unsweetened almond milk (or milk of choice)
- 1/2 frozen banana
- 1/4 cup of spinach
- 1 tbsp chia seeds
- 1/4 tsp ground ginger (optional)
- Pinch of cinnamon

Toppings (choose 3-4):

Chopped fresh berries, sliced banana or apple, Chopped nuts, Shredded coconut, Granola, Drizzle of almond butter or honey (optional)

Instructions

1. Tenderize your fresh beetroot through either steaming or roasting before chopping it.
2. Blend all the smoothie base ingredients together in a blender until they are mixed to a smooth and creamy texture.
3. Pour the smoothie into a bowl and top it with your favorite toppings artistically and vibrantly.

Nutrition per serving:

Calories: 300 Fat: 10g Carbs: 35g
Protein: 7g

Fruity Greens Smoothie Bowl

Prep time: 10 minutes Cook time: None
Servings: 1

Ingredients

Smoothie Base:

- 1 cup of unsweetened almond milk
- 1/2 cup of chopped kale or spinach
- 1/2 frozen mango
- 1/4 frozen pineapple
- 1/4 avocado
- 1 scoop plant-based protein powder (optional)
- 1/4 tsp ground ginger (optional)
- Pinch of cinnamon

Instructions

1. Clean and roughly cut the spinach or kale.
2. Mix all of the ingredients for the smoothie base; process until smooth and creamy.
3. Transfer the blended drink to a bowl. Add your preferred toppings on top in a vibrant and imaginative design.

Nutrition per serving

Calories: 300 Fat: 10g Carbs: 35g
Protein: 15g

Fruity Yogurt Bowl

Prep time: 5 minutes Cook time: None
Servings: 1

Ingredients

- 1 cup of plain Greek yogurt
- 1/2 cup of chopped fresh fruit of your choice
- 1/4 cup of chopped nuts or seeds
- 1/4 tsp ground cinnamon or ginger (optional)
- Drizzle of honey or maple syrup (optional)
- Fresh mint leaves (optional)

Instructions

1. Choose your fruit and wash and cut it.
2. Yogurt is spooned into a bowl. Add chopped fruit, nuts or seeds, cinnamon or ginger (if used), and (optional) a drizzle of honey or maple syrup.
3. Add a few fresh mint leaves (optional) for a cool touch.

Nutrition per serving

Calories: 250 Fat: 10g Carbs: 25g
Protein: 20g

Granola Yogurt Bowl

Prep time: 5 minutes Servings: 1

Ingredients

- 1 cup of plain Greek yogurt
- 1/4 cup of homemade or store-bought granola
- 1/2 cup of chopped fresh fruit of your choice
- 1/4 cup of nuts or seeds
- Pinch of cinnamon or ground ginger (optional)
- Drizzle of honey or maple syrup (optional)
- Fresh mint leaves (optional)

Instructions

1. Pick a Greek yogurt that is simple and unsweetened for maximum nutritional benefits.
2. Choose your fruit and wash and cut it. For crunch and extra flavor, gently toast the nuts or seeds (optional).
3. Yogurt is spooned into a bowl. Arrange the fruit, granola, nuts, seeds, and, if desired, cinnamon and ginger in layers.
4. For a refreshing touch, sprinkle in some fresh mint leaves and drizzle with honey or maple syrup (optional).

Nutrition per serving

Calories: 300 Fat: 10g Carbs: 30g
Protein: 20g

Chicken & Fruit Salad

Prep time: 15 minutes Cook time: 10-15 minutes Servings: 2

Ingredients

For the salad:

- 2 boneless, skinless chicken breasts, grilled or baked
- 1 cup of chopped mixed greens (spinach, romaine, kale)
- 1/2 cup of chopped fresh fruit of your choice (berries, mango, pineapple, grapes)
- 1/4 cup of chopped cucumber
- 1/4 cup of crumbled feta cheese (optional)
- 1/4 cup of chopped walnuts or pecans
- Fresh herbs for garnish (optional: mint, basil, parsley)

For the dressing

- 2 tbsp olive oil
- 1 tbsp Dijon mustard
- 1 tbsp honey
- 1 tbsp apple cider vinegar
- Pinch of salt and pepper

Instructions

1. Cook the chicken breasts well on the grill or in the oven. Allow to cool slightly before slicing or shredding into small pieces.
2. Toss the greens, diced fruit, cucumber, feta cheese (if using), pecans or walnuts, and optional seasonings in a big bowl.
3. Mix the olive oil, Dijon mustard, honey, apple cider vinegar, salt, and pepper in a small bowl.
4. After making the dressing, drizzle it over the salad and gently toss to mix. Serve right away after adding the sliced or shredded chicken on top.

Nutrition per serving

Calories: 400 Fat: 20g Carbs: 30g Protein: 12g

Chicken, Jicama & Carrot Salad

Prep time: 15 minutes Cook time: 10-15 minutes Servings: 2-3

Ingredients

For the salad:

- 2 boneless, skinless chicken breasts, grilled or baked
- 2 cups of jicama, peeled and matchsticks
- 2 cups of carrots, peeled and matchsticks
- 1 red bell pepper, thinly sliced (optional)

- 1/2 red onion, thinly sliced (optional)
- 1/4 cup of chopped fresh cilantro
- 1/4 cup of chopped fresh parsley
- 1/4 cup of sunflower seeds
- Fresh lime wedges for garnish

For the dressing:

- 2 tbsp olive oil
- 2 tbsp fresh lime juice
- 1 tsp Dijon mustard
- 1/2 tsp honey
- Pinch of salt and pepper

Instructions

1. Cook the chicken breasts well on the grill or in the oven. Allow to cool slightly before slicing or shredding into small pieces.
2. Peel and finely chop the carrots and jicama. Cut the red onion and bell pepper thinly (optional). Finely chop the parsley and cilantro.
3. The cooked chicken, jicama, carrots, bell pepper, red onion, cilantro, parsley, and sunflower seeds should all be mixed in a big dish.
4. Mix the olive oil, lime juice, Dijon mustard, honey, salt, and pepper in a small bowl.
5. After making the dressing, drizzle it over the salad and gently toss to mix. To add a tangy and refreshing touch, serve immediately with fresh lime wedges.

Nutrition per serving

Calories: 400 Fat: 20g Carbs: 25g Protein: 35g

Steak & Veggie Salad

Prep time: 15 minutes Cook time: 15-20 minutes Servings: 1

Ingredients

For the salad:

- 1 boneless ribeye steak trimmed and seasoned
- 1 cup of mixed greens (spinach, romaine, kale)
- 1 cup of roasted vegetables
- 1/2 avocado, sliced
- 1/4 cup of crumbled feta cheese (optional)
- 1/4 cup of chopped walnuts or pecans
- Fresh herbs for garnish

For the dressing:

- 2 tbsp olive oil
- 2 tbsp balsamic vinegar
- 1 tsp Dijon mustard
- 1/2 tsp honey
- Pinch of salt and pepper

Instructions

1. Cook the steak till the doneness you choose. After allowing it to rest for five minutes, thinly cut it against the grain.
2. Turn the oven on to 400°F or 200°C. Mix salt, pepper, and olive oil with chopped veggies. Place

onto a baking sheet, then roast for 15 to 20 minutes or until soft and beginning to turn golden.

3. The roasted veggies, avocado slices, feta cheese (if used), walnuts or pecans, and your preferred herbs (optional) should all be mixed in a big dish.

4. Mix the olive oil, balsamic vinegar, Dijon mustard, honey, salt, and pepper in a small bowl.

5. After making the dressing, drizzle it over the salad and gently toss to mix. Place the cut steak on top and serve right away.

Nutrition per serving

Calories: 500 Fat: 25g Carbs: 25g Protein: 45g

Salmon, Orange & Beet Salad

Prep time: 15 minutes Cook time: 15-20 minutes Servings: 1-2

Ingredients

For the salad:

- 4 oz boneless, skinless salmon fillet, baked or grilled
- 1 cup of mixed greens
- 1 medium beet, roasted and cubed
- 1 medium orange, segmented
- 1/4 cup of crumbled feta cheese (optional)
- 1/4 cup of chopped walnuts or pecans
- Fresh herbs for garnish

For the dressing:

- 2 tbsp olive oil
- 2 tbsp orange juice
- 1 tbsp balsamic vinegar
- 1 tsp Dijon mustard
- 1/2 tsp honey
- Pinch of salt and pepper

Instructions

1. The salmon fillet should be cooked thoroughly, whether baked or grilled. After allowing it to cool slightly, break it up into little pieces.

2. Adjust oven temperature to 400°F (200°C) if using fresh beets. When the beet is soft, roast it with foil for 45 to 60 minutes; after letting it cool, peel and cube.

3. Add the cooked salmon, roasted beet cubes, orange segments, feta cheese (if using), walnuts or pecans, and your preferred herbs (optional) to a large bowl.

4. Mix the olive oil, orange juice, honey, Dijon mustard, balsamic vinegar, and salt and pepper in a small bowl.

5. After making the dressing, drizzle it over the salad and gently toss to mix. Serve right away.

Nutrition per serving:

Calories: 400 Fat: 20g Carbs: 25g Protein: 35g

Salmon & Veggie Salad

Prep time: 15 minutes Cook time: 15-20 minutes Servings: 1-2

Ingredients

For the salad:

- 4 oz boneless, skinless salmon fillet, baked or grilled
- 1 cup of mixed greens
- 1 cup of roasted vegetables
- 1/2 avocado, sliced
- 1/4 cup of chopped fresh dill
- 1/4 cup of sunflower seeds
- Fresh lemon wedges for garnish

For the dressing:

- 2 tbsp olive oil
- 2 tbsp lemon juice
- 1 tsp Dijon mustard
- 1/2 tsp honey
- Pinch of salt and pepper

Instructions

1. Bake or grill the salmon fillet till it is cooked. Wait and let it cool before flaking into small pieces you can chew.
2. Preheat oven to 400°F (200°C). Chop vegetables, then toss them in olive oil, salt and pepper. Spread on a baking sheet and roast for 15-20 minutes until tender and slightly browned.
3. Mix greens, roasted vegetables, avocado slices, fresh dill, sunflower seeds, and your chosen herbs (optional) in a large bowl.
4. In a small bowl, beat the olive oil, lemon juice, Dijon mustard, honey salt, and pepper.
5. Drizzle the prepared dressing over the salad; gently toss to mix. Top with the flaked salmon and serve with wedges of fresh lemon for a citrusy touch.

Nutrition per serving

Calories: 400 Fat: 20g Carbs: 25g Protein: 35g

Tuna & Egg Salad

Prep time: 10 minutes Cook time: 10 minutes Servings: 1-2

Ingredients

- 1 (5 oz) can tuna packed in water, drained
- 2 hard-boiled eggs, chopped
- 1/2 cup of chopped celery
- 1/4 avocado, mashed
- 1 tbsp Greek yogurt (plain, unsweetened)
- 1 tsp Dijon mustard
- 1/2 tbsp lemon juice
- Pinch of salt and pepper
- Fresh herbs for garnish (optional: dill, parsley)

Instructions

1. Drain tuna and flake it in a bowl with a fork.
2. Remove the shell and chop hard-boiled eggs.

3. In a bowl, flake the tuna, chop the eggs, and add celery, mashed avocado, Greek yogurt, Dijon mustard, lemon juice, salt, and pepper. Mix gently until everything is well mixed.
4. If it seems too thick, add more yogurt or some water.
5. Eat it alone as a tuna & egg salad or serve on lettuce leaves, whole wheat bread, or crackers. Additionally, you may garnish it with fresh herbs for an extra touch of flavor.

Nutrition per serving

Calories: 300 Fat: 15g Carbs: 10g Protein: 25g

Shrimp & Greens Salad

Prep time: 15 minutes Cook time: 5-7 minutes Servings: 2

Ingredients:

For the salad:

- 1/2 lb. shrimp
- 4 cups of mixed greens
- 1/2 avocado, sliced
- 1/2 cup of cherry tomatoes, halved
- 1/4 cup of chopped red onion (optional)
- 1/4 cup of crumbled feta cheese (optional)
- Fresh cilantro leaves for garnish

For the dressing

- 2 tbsp olive oil
- 2 tbsp lime juice
- 1 tsp Dijon mustard
- 1/2 tsp honey
- 1/4 cup of chopped fresh cilantro
- Pinch of salt and pepper

Instructions

1. Shrimp should be sautéed or grilled until they turn slightly pink and are thoroughly cooked. Cook them sufficiently, then cut them into sizes that can be bitten.
2. In a big bowl, mix spinach, avocado slices, cherry tomatoes, and onion (no need if you choose) and feta cheese (if desired).
3. Mix olive oil, lime juice, Dijon mustard, honey, chopped cilantro, salt, and pepper in a small dish.
4. Pour the prepared dressing on the salad, then stir it smoothly. Place shrimp on top of it, then decorate with cilantro leaves.

Nutrition per serving

Calories: 400 Fat: 20g Carbs: 25g Protein: 35g

Shrimp & Tomato Salad

Prep time: 15 minutes Cook time: 5-7 minutes Servings: 2

Ingredients

For the salad:

- 1/2 lb. shrimp
- 2 cups of chopped tomatoes

- 1 cup of chopped cucumber
- 1/4 cup of chopped red onion (optional)
- 1/4 cup of crumbled feta cheese (optional)
- 1/4 cup of chopped fresh parsley
- 1/4 cup of chopped fresh basil
- Fresh lemon wedges for garnish

For the dressing:

- 4 tbsp plain Greek yogurt
- 1 tbsp olive oil
- 1 tsp lemon juice
- 1/2 tsp dried oregano
- Pinch of salt and pepper

Instructions

1. The shrimp should be cooked through and slightly pink by either sautéing or grilling. After that, let it cool a bit, then cut it into bite-size pieces.
2. Chopped tomatoes, cucumber, red onion (optional), feta cheese (optional), parsley, and basil are all mixed in one big bowl.
3. Greek yogurt, olive oil, lemon juice, oregano, salt, and pepper should be whisked in a small bowl.
4. Toss gently to mix after drizzling the prepared dressing over the salad. Top with the cooked shrimp and garnish with fresh lemon wedges.

Nutrition per serving:

Calories: 350 Fat: 15g Carbs: 20g Protein: 35g

Berries & Watermelon Salad

Prep time: 10 minutes Cook time: None Servings: 2

Ingredients:

For the salad:

- 2 cups of cubed seedless watermelon
- 1 cup of mixed berries
- 1/4 cup of chopped fresh mint leaves
- 1/4 cup of crumbled feta cheese (optional)

For the dressing:

- 2 tbsp olive oil
- 1 tbsp lime juice
- 1 tsp honey
- Pinch of salt and pepper

Instructions:

1. Cut the watermelon into small pieces and wash it. Wash the berries carefully.
2. The mixture includes watermelon, berries, and mint leaves.
3. Blend olive oil, lime juice, honey, salt, and pepper in another bowl.
4. Pour the prepared dressing on top of the salad and gently mix it. Optionally, sprinkle crumbled feta cheese on top and serve immediately.

Nutrition per serving:

Calories: 250 Fat: 10g Carbs: 30g
Protein: 10g

Rocket & Orange Salad

Prep time: 10 minutes. Servings: 1-2

Ingredients

For the salad:

- 2 cups of arugula (rocket)
- 1 large orange, segmented
- 1/2 avocado, thinly sliced
- 1/4 cup of chopped walnuts
- Fresh herbs for garnish

For the dressing:

- 2 tbsp olive oil
- 2 tbsp orange juice
- 1 tbsp balsamic vinegar
- 1 tsp Dijon mustard
- 1/2 tsp honey
- Pinch of salt and pepper

Instructions

1. Segment and peel the orange, ensuring you eliminate the white membrane to make the taste less bitter.
2. Avocado slices, orange segments, walnuts, and arugula should be mixed in a big bowl.
3. Mix olive oil, orange juice, balsamic vinegar, Dijon mustard, honey, salt, and pepper in a small bowl, then whisk together.
4. Then drizzle the prepared dressing over the salad and toss gently to

mix. Garnish with fresh herbs (optional) and serve immediately.

Nutrition per serving:

Calories: 300 Fat: 20g Carbs: 25g
Protein: 10g

Mango & Bell Pepper Salad

Prep time: 15 minutes Cook time: None
Servings: 2

Ingredients

For the salad:

- 1 ripe mango, cubed
- 1 cup of chopped bell peppers
- 1/2 avocado, thinly sliced
- 1/4 cup of chopped red onion (optional)
- Fresh cilantro leaves for garnish

For the dressing:

- 2 tbsp olive oil
- 2 tbsp lime juice
- 1 tsp honey
- 1/4 tsp Dijon mustard
- 1/4 cup of chopped fresh cilantro
- Pinch of salt and pepper

Instructions

1. The ripe mango is supposed to be peeled and cubed.
2. Next, you will wash the bell peppers and remove the seeds before you dice them into small pieces that can easily be bitten.

3. Mix mango cubes, bell pepper, avocado slices, and red onion (optional) in a large bowl.
4. Mix olive oil, lime juice, honey, Dijon mustard, chopped cilantro, salt, and pepper in a small bowl to prepare the dressing.
5. The salad should be prepared by drizzling the dressing and then gently mixing. Add fresh cilantro leaves to garnish it, and it is ready for serving.

Nutrition per serving:

Calories: 350 Fat: 20g Carbs: 25g Protein: 10g

Beet, Carrot & Apple Salad

Prep time: 15 minutes Cook time: 45-60 minutes Servings: 2-3

Ingredients

For the salad:

- 2 medium beets, roasted and cubed
- 2 large carrots, peeled and grated
- 1 medium apple, cored and chopped
- 1/4 cup of chopped walnuts or pecans
- Fresh herbs for garnish (optional: parsley, dill, chives)

For the dressing:

- 2 tbsp olive oil
- 2 tbsp balsamic vinegar
- 1 tsp Dijon mustard
- 1/2 tsp honey
- Pinch of salt and pepper

Instructions

1. If you use fresh beets, preheat oven to 400°F (200°C). Cover them with foil and roast them for 45-60 minutes until tender. Afterward, allow it to cool, peel off the skin, and cut it into pieces.
2. Wash the carrots before peeling them, then grate them using a box grater or food processor.
3. Wash, remove the core, and dice the apple into bite-sized bits.
4. Mix roasted beet cubes, grated carrots, chopped apples, and walnuts/pecans in a mixing bowl.
5. Whisk together oil, v, vinegar, mustard, honey, salt, and pepper in another small bowl.
6. Pour prepared dressing over the salad, then gently toss it all together. Add herbs on top if desired, but consume the salad immediately.

Nutrition per serving:

Calories: 300 Fat: 15g Carbs: 25g Protein: 10g

Tomato & Mozzarella Salad

Prep time: 10 minutes. Servings: 1-2

Ingredients

For the salad:

- 2 large ripe tomatoes, sliced
- 1 ball fresh mozzarella cheese, sliced or torn
- 1/2 cup of fresh basil leaves, torn
- Extra virgin olive oil for drizzling
- Sea salt and freshly ground black pepper, to taste

Optional additions:

- Balsamic glaze
- Capers
- Red onion, thinly sliced
- Fresh oregano leaves

Instructions

1. Choose fully ripe tomato tomatoes with bright colors, good sweet-acid taste, and the best flavor. Heirlooms have a complex flavor.
2. You can overlap the tomato slices on a platter. They should be then smothered in sliced or torn mozzarella cheese.
3. Some fresh basil leaves may just be scattered over it.
4. Afterward, drizzle some extra virgin olive oil lavishly as you season it with sea salt and freshly ground black pepper to your liking.
5. For a different taste with balsamic vinegar, pour balsamic glaze all over them. Additional flavors and crispness may come from capers, red onion rounds, or oregano sprigs.

Nutrition per serving:

Calories: 300 Fat: 20g Carbs: 20g Protein: 20g

Collard Greens & Seeds Salad

Prep time: 15 minutes Cook time: 5 minutes Servings: 2-3

Ingredients:

For the salad:

- 4 cups of chopped collard greens
- 1/2 cup of sunflower seeds, toasted
- 1/4 cup of dried cranberries
- 1/4 cup of crumbled feta cheese (optional)
- Fresh herbs for garnish

For the dressing:

- 2 tbsp olive oil
- 2 tbsp lemon juice
- 1 tsp honey
- Pinch of salt and pepper

Instructions

1. If you are using fresh greens, rinse and remove tough stems from collard greens, then chop them finely or rub them with a bit of olive oil to tenderize.
2. Toast dry sunflower seeds in a pan over medium heat for 5-7 minutes,

stirring occasionally until they become fragrant and light-browned.

3. Mix the chopped collard greens, toasted sunflower seeds, cranberries, and feta cheese (optional) in a large bowl.
4. Whisk the olive oil, lemon juice, honey, salt, and pepper in a small bowl together.
5. Pour prepared dressing over the salad and toss gently. You may decorate it with optional fresh herbs for immediate consumption.

Nutrition per serving:

Calories: 300 Fat: 20g Carbs: 25g
Protein: 10g

Carrot & Radish Salad

Prep time: 10 minutes Servings: 2-3

Ingredients

For the salad:

- 2 large carrots, grated
- 1 bunch radishes, trimmed and thinly sliced
- 1/2 avocado, thinly sliced
- 1/4 cup of chopped fresh dill
- Freshly ground black pepper, to taste

For the dressing:

- 2 tbsp olive oil
- 2 tbsp lemon juice
- 1/2 tsp Dijon mustard
- Pinch of salt and pepper

Instructions

1. Peel and wash carrots and grate them with a box grater or food processor.
2. Slice radishes into thin, trim pieces.
3. Mix grated carrots, sliced radishes, avocado slices, and chopped dill in a large bowl. Add freshly ground black pepper to taste.
4. Whisk olive oil with lemon juice, Dijon mustard, salt, and pepper in a small bowl.
5. Drizzle the prepared dressing across the salad and mix gently. The freshest flavor can be enjoyed instantly.

Nutrition per serving

Calories: 250 Fat: 15g Carbs: 20g
Protein: 10g

Lentil & Apple Salad

Prep time: 15 minutes Cook time: 20-30 minutes Servings: 2-3

Ingredients

For the salad:

- 1 cup of cooked lentils
- 1 large apple, cored and chopped
- 1/2 cup of chopped celery
- 1/4 cup of crumbled feta cheese
- 1/4 cup of chopped walnuts or pecans
- Fresh herbs for garnish

For the dressing:

- 2 tbsp olive oil
- 2 tbsp apple cider vinegar or Dijon mustard
- 1 tsp honey
- Pinch of salt and pepper

Instructions:

1. Rinse and cook the lentils using dry ones according to package instructions. Aim for al dente texture.
2. The apple is going to be washed, cored, and chopped. The celery will be sliced thinly after washing it.
3. Mix the cooked lentils, chopped apple, celery, feta cheese, and walnuts/pecans in a large bowl.
4. Mix the olive oil with Dijon mustard or apple cider vinegar, salt and pepper, and honey in a small bowl.
5. The prepared dressing should be drizzled over the salad before gently tossing them together. You may garnish with fresh herbs (optional) and enjoy immediately.

Nutrition per serving:

Calories: 350 Fat: 20g Carbs: 30g
Protein: 20g

Turkey & Veggies Soup

Prep time: 15 minutes Cook time: 30 minutes Servings: 4-6

Ingredients:

For the soup:

- 1 tbsp olive oil
- 1/2 onion, chopped
- 2 cloves garlic, minced
- 1 lb. ground turkey (90% lean or higher)
- 2 carrots, peeled and diced
- 2 stalks celery, diced
- 1 zucchini, diced
- 1 cup of frozen corn
- 6 cups of low-sodium chicken or vegetable broth
- 1 (14.5 oz) can of diced tomatoes, undrained
- 1 tbsp chopped fresh parsley
- Salt and pepper to taste

Optional additions:

- 1 bay leaf
- 1/2 tsp dried thyme
- Chopped kale or spinach
- Cooked brown rice or quinoa

Instructions

1. The olive oil is heated over medium heat in a large pot or Dutch oven.
2. Add the chopped onion and sauté until softened, about 3-4 minutes. Stir in the minced garlic and cook for another minute until it becomes fragrant.
3. The ground turkey should be added to the pot and cooked well while breaking it up with a spoon. Drain off any fat.
4. Stir in diced zucchini, carrots, and celery. Let them cook for 5-7 minutes till slightly softened.
5. Now add chicken or vegetable broth and diced tomatoes with their juices. Bring to a boil, reduce heat, and simmer for around fifteen minutes.
6. Simmer for an additional 5 minutes while stirring in frozen corn and parsley. The corn will heat through.
7. Salt and pepper should be adjusted to taste. Serve hot, garnished with more parsley or a dollop of plain Greek yogurt (optional).

Nutrition per serving:

Calories: 350 Fat: 15g Carbs: 35g
Protein: 30g

Ground Turkey & Cabbage Soup

Prep time: 15 minutes Cook time: 30-35 minutes Servings: 4-6

Ingredients

For the soup:

- 1 tbsp olive oil
- 1 onion, chopped
- 2 cloves garlic, minced
- 1 lb. ground turkey (90% lean or higher)
- 1/2 head cabbage, thinly sliced
- 2 carrots, peeled and diced
- 4 cups of low-sodium chicken or vegetable broth
- 1 (14.5 oz) can of diced tomatoes, undrained
- 1 tbsp chopped fresh parsley
- 1 tsp dried thyme
- 1/2 tsp dried oregano
- Pinch of red pepper flakes (optional)
- Salt and pepper to taste

Optional additions:

- 1 bay leaf
- Handful of chopped celery
- 1 cup of chopped mushrooms
- 1 tsp lemon juice
- Cooked brown rice or quinoa

Instructions

1. Heat the olive oil over medium heat in a large pot or Dutch oven.
2. Sauté for three to four minutes until onions are softened. Stir in garlic and cook until it becomes fragrant for about one minute.
3. Add turkey and cook while stirring with a spoon to break it apart till browned. Remove excess fat.
4. Then, add the sliced cabbage and diced carrots. Cook them for five to seven minutes so the cabbage is slightly wilted.
5. Put in chicken or vegetable broth, tomatoes with juice, herbs, and spices (thyme, oregano, red pepper flakes). Bring to a boil, then reduce heat and simmer between 20 and 25 minutes until cabbage and carrots are tender.
6. Salt and pepper may be added for taste. Optionally stir in some chopped parsley or lemon juice. Serve hot together with extra parsley leaves or plain Greek yogurt on top of it.

Nutrition per serving:

Calories: 300 Fat: 15g Carbs: 25g Protein: 25g

Beef & Lentil Soup

Prep time: 15 minutes Cook time: 45 minutes Servings: 4-6

Ingredients

For the soup:

- 1 tbsp olive oil
- 1 onion, chopped
- 2 cloves garlic, minced

- 1 lb. lean stew beef, cut into bite-sized pieces
- 1 carrot, peeled and diced
- 1 stalk celery, diced
- 1/2 cup of green beans, trimmed and chopped
- 1/2 cup of brown lentils, rinsed
- 4 cups of low-sodium beef or vegetable broth
- 1 (14.5 oz) can of diced tomatoes, undrained
- 1 tsp dried thyme
- 1/2 tsp dried rosemary
- Pinch of red pepper flakes (optional)
- Salt and pepper to taste

Optional additions:

- 1 bay leaf
- 1 cup of chopped mushrooms
- Handful of chopped kale or spinach
- Cooked brown rice or quinoa

Instructions

1. Warm olive oil in a large pot or Dutch oven on medium heat.
2. Cook the onion until it is sautéed and softened for 3-4 minutes. The minced garlic is added, which should be cooked for another minute to give out its fragrance.
3. Put in the stew beef and brown all sides. If there's any extra fat in it, it should be drained off.
4. Mix diced carrots, celery, green beans, and brown lentils. Allow them to cook for about 5-7 minutes so that even vegetables become soft.

5. Add diced tomatoes to that beef or vegetable broth with their juice, herbs, and spices (thyme, rosemary, red pepper flakes). Let it boil, then reduce the heat and simmer for 30-35 minutes until the lentils are tender.
6. Put salt and pepper to taste. Add chopped kale or spinach during the last few minutes of cooking (optional). Serve hot topped with plain Greek yogurt (optional).

Nutrition per serving:

Calories: 350 Fat: 20g Carbs: 35g Protein: 35g

Beef & Carrot Stew

Prep time: 15 minutes Cook time: 1 hour Servings: 4-6

Ingredients

For the stew:

- 1 tbsp olive oil
- 1 onion, chopped
- 2 cloves garlic, minced
- 1 lb. beef chuck roast, cut into bite-sized pieces
- 1/2 tsp dried thyme
- 1/2 tsp dried rosemary
- Salt and pepper to taste
- 4 cups of low-sodium beef or vegetable broth
- 1 (14.5 oz) can of diced tomatoes, undrained
- 3 large carrots, peeled and roughly chopped

- 2 parsnips, peeled and roughly chopped
- 1 bay leaf (optional)

Optional additions:

- 1 tbsp tomato paste
- 1 cup of chopped celery
- 1 cup of chopped mushrooms
- Handful of chopped fresh parsley
- Cooked brown rice or quinoa

Instructions

1. The olive oil should be heated over medium heat in a large pot or Dutch oven.
2. After 3-4 minutes, add the minced onion and cook until soft. The finely chopped garlic follows, cooked for just a minute to give out its fragrance.
3. The beef has to be seasoned with thyme, rosemary, salt, and pepper before adding it to the pot so it is brown on all sides. It would be drained from any fat remaining.
4. Beef broth, tomatoes diced with their juices, and bay leaf (optional) are added next. Bring this mixture to a boil and simmer for 30 minutes with reduced heat.
5. Also, add in the parsnips and carrots, which are chopped. If available, mushrooms and celery can also be used while simmering for around 20-25 minutes or until beef is cooked and vegetables turn tender.
6. For a thicker consistency, if you prefer, stir in tomato paste (optional). Add more salt and pepper if necessary.
7. Garnish this dish with freshly cut parsley (optional) while still hot, and serve it with brown rice or cooked quinoa.

Nutrition per serving:

Calories: 400 Fat: 20g Carbs: 35g Protein: 35g

Salmon & Shrimp Stew

Prep time: 15 minutes Cook time: 30 minutes Servings: 4-6

Ingredients

For the stew:

- 1 tbsp olive oil
- 1 onion, chopped
- 2 cloves garlic, minced
- 1/2 red bell pepper, chopped
- 1/2 green bell pepper, chopped
- 1 zucchini, diced
- 1 cup of chopped cherry tomatoes
- 4 cups of low-sodium chicken or vegetable broth
- 1 (14.5 oz) can of diced tomatoes, undrained
- 1 bay leaf
- 1/2 tsp dried thyme
- 1/4 tsp dried oregano
- Pinch of saffron (optional)
- Salt and pepper to taste
- 12 oz. skinless salmon fillets cut into bite-sized pieces

- 1/2 lb. raw shrimp, peeled and deveined

Optional additions:

- 1 tbsp tomato paste
- Handful of chopped fresh parsley
- Cooked brown rice or quinoa

Instructions

1. Warm olive oil over medium heat in a large pot or Dutch oven.
2. Put in the chopped onion and sauté for 3-4 minutes until soft. Add the minced garlic and cook for another minute till you can smell its aroma.
3. Cook for 5-7 minutes up to a tender point of the vegetables when they are added into the pot with chopped bell peppers and zucchini.
4. Pour chicken or vegetable broth, diced tomatoes, herbs such as thyme and oregano, bay leaf, and saffron (if you want). Let it boil on high heat, then simmer on low heat for 10 minutes.
5. Salt and pepper the broth accordingly. Stir the salmon chunks gently while just done (flaky and opaque) for about 5-7 minutes.
6. Again, put it on low flame and add peeled shrimp, which has been deveined. Cook till they turn pink as if finished off completely, about 2-3 minutes more.
7. Another option is tomato paste to thicken the soup. Finally, serve it with some brown rice or quinoa after adding parsley, which is fresh but has been chopped into small pieces on top of it.

Nutrition per serving:

Calories: 350 Fat: 15g Carbs: 30g Protein: 35g

Mushroom & Kale Stew

Prep time: 15 minutes Cook time: 30 minutes Servings: 4-6

Ingredients

For the stew:

- 1 tbsp olive oil
- 1 onion, chopped
- 2 cloves garlic, minced
- 1 lb. mixed mushrooms sliced
- 1 large carrot, peeled and diced
- 1/2 cup of chopped celery
- 1 (14.5 oz) can of diced tomatoes, undrained
- 4 cups of low-sodium vegetable broth
- 1 (13.5 oz) can unsweetened coconut milk
- 1/2 tsp dried thyme
- 1/4 tsp dried rosemary
- Pinch of red pepper flakes (optional)
- Salt and pepper to taste
- 4 cups of chopped kale

Optional additions:

- 1 cup of cooked brown rice or quinoa
- Handful of chopped fresh parsley

Instructions

1. Over medium heat, heat olive oil in a large pot or Dutch oven.
2. Until it softens, allow the chopped onion to sauté for about 3 minutes. Cook minced garlic in and stir it for one minute longer until it becomes aromatic.
3. Soften the mushrooms for 5-7 minutes until they are browned and slightly softened.
4. Dice tomatoes with their juice before including them in the broth. Stir in the diced carrots and chopped celery, then cook for a few more minutes until they get tender. Bring to a boil and simmer over reduced heat for ten minutes with vegetable broth.
5. Add the thyme, rosemary, red pepper flakes (optional) into the coconut milk and mix well. Taste with salt and pepper. Continue cooking for about five more minutes.
6. The kale will be gently folded and taken off after two or three minutes when it has wilted and become tender.
7. Garnish with parsley that is freshly chopped, but this is optional. Serve hot. Also, you can enjoy this meal with quinoa or brown rice, which has been cooked beforehand.

Nutrition per serving:

Calories: 300 Fat: 15g Carbs: 30g Protein: 15g

Mixed Veggie Stew

Prep time: 15 minutes Cook time: 30 minutes Servings: 4-6

Ingredients

For the stew:

- 1 tbsp olive oil
- 1 onion, chopped
- 2 cloves garlic, minced
- 1 stalk celery, chopped
- 1 carrot, peeled and diced
- 1 zucchini, diced
- 1 bell pepper (any color), chopped
- 1 cup of green beans, trimmed and chopped
- 1 (14.5 oz) can of diced tomatoes, undrained
- 4 cups of low-sodium vegetable broth
- 1 bay leaf
- 1/2 tsp dried thyme
- 1/4 tsp dried oregano
- Pinch of red pepper flakes (optional)
- Salt and pepper to taste

Optional additions:

- 1 tbsp tomato paste
- Handful of chopped fresh parsley
- Cooked brown rice or quinoa

Instructions

1. A large pot or Dutch oven should be heated over medium heat with olive oil.
2. Chopped onion is added and then sautéed for 3-4 minutes until it gets

soft. Minced garlic is stirred in and cooked further for one more minute till it smells good.

3. Afterward, chopped celery and diced carrots are mixed in. They are cooked for 5-7 minutes to soften a bit.
4. In addition, add zucchini, bell pepper, and green beans. Cook this mixture for about five more minutes until it becomes softer.
5. Tomato juice with its dice, vegetable broth, bay leaf, herbs (thyme, oregano), and red pepper flakes (optional) must be brought to a boil. Then, decrease the fire and let it simmer for 15 to 20 minutes or until vegetables become tender.
6. For thicker consistency, tomato paste can also be stirred in (optional) and salted and peppered according to your taste.
7. Garnish with chopped fresh parsley (optional), and serve hot with cooked brown rice or quinoa to make a more substantial meal.

Nutrition per serving:

Calories: 250 Fat: 10g Carbs: 30g Protein: 10g

Quinoa & Veggie Stew

Prep time: 15 minutes Cook time: 30 minutes Servings: 4-6

Ingredients:

For the stew:

- 1 tbsp olive oil
- 1 onion, chopped
- 2 cloves garlic, minced
- 1 stalk celery, chopped
- 1 carrot, peeled and diced
- 1 zucchini, diced
- 1 bell pepper (any color), chopped
- 1 cup of chopped broccoli florets
- 1 (14.5 oz) can of diced tomatoes, undrained
- 4 cups of low-sodium vegetable broth
- 1 cup of rinsed quinoa
- 1 bay leaf
- 1/2 tsp dried thyme
- 1/4 tsp dried oregano
- Pinch of red pepper flakes (optional)
- Salt and pepper to taste

Optional additions:

- 1 tbsp tomato paste
- Handful of chopped fresh parsley
- Cooked brown rice (for an additional serving option)

Instructions

1. Olive oil should be heated in a large pan or Dutch oven over medium heat.
2. Sauté the chopped onion for about 3-4 minutes until it becomes soft. After that, stir the minced garlic and fry for one more minute until it smells nice.
3. Celery should be chopped and mixed with finely chopped carrots. Then, cook them on low heat for

approximately five to seven minutes until they become tender.

4. Zucchini, bell pepper, and broccoli florets should also be added and cooked for another five minutes to make them slightly softer.

5. Add diced tomatoes with their juice, vegetable broth, washed quinoa, bay leaf, herbs (thyme and oregano), and red pepper flakes (optional). It is brought to a boil before reducing the heat to simmer for at least 20 minutes or when the quinoa is cooked and all vegetables are tender.

6. Tomato paste can be stirred in to increase its thickness if desired. For taste, add salt as well as pepper.

7. It can then be garnished with freshly chopped parsley before serving hot. One may also choose to eat it alone or accompany it with brown rice prepared elsewhere to get enhanced texture together with carbohydrates.

Nutrition per serving:

Calories: 350 Fat: 10g Carbs: 40g
Protein: 20g

Salmon & Cabbage Soup

Prep time: 15 minutes Cook time: 30 minutes Servings: 4-6

Ingredients

For the soup:

- 1 tbsp olive oil
- 1 onion, chopped
- 2 cloves garlic, minced
- 1/2 head cabbage, thinly sliced
- 2 carrots, peeled and diced
- 4 cups of low-sodium chicken or vegetable broth
- 1 (14.5 oz) can of diced tomatoes, undrained
- 1 bay leaf
- 1/2 tsp dried thyme
- 1/4 tsp dried oregano
- Pinch of red pepper flakes (optional)
- Salt and pepper to taste
- 12 oz. skinless salmon fillets cut into bite-sized pieces

Optional additions:

- 1 tbsp tomato paste
- Handful of chopped fresh parsley
- Cooked brown rice or quinoa

Instructions

1. Heat the olive oil in a big pot or Dutch oven on medium heat.

2. The onion is sautéed for 3-4 minutes until it turns soft. Garlic should be mixed with it and cooked for another minute till fragrant.

3. Thinly slice cabbage and add some diced carrots. Let them cook for at least five to seven minutes until slightly soft.

4. Put in chicken (or vegetable) broth, the juice of diced tomatoes, bay leaf, herbs (thyme and oregano), and red pepper flakes (optional). Bring to a boil, then reduce heat to simmer for 15 minutes.

5. Lastly, season the broth with salt and pepper. The salmon pieces are gently stirred while cooking for 5-7 minutes and removed just when cooked through (flaky white inside).

6. Tomato paste can be added to make the soup thicker (optional). Add chopped fresh parsley if desired, and serve hot with brown rice or quinoa.

Nutrition per serving:

Calories: 350 Fat: 15g Carbs: 30g Protein: 35g

Shrimp & Mushroom Soup

Prep time: 15 minutes Cook time: 30 minutes Servings: 4-6

Ingredients

For the soup:

- 1 tbsp olive oil
- 1 onion, chopped
- 2 cloves garlic, minced
- 1/2 red bell pepper, chopped
- 1/2 green bell pepper, chopped
- 1 zucchini, diced
- 1 cup of sliced shiitake mushrooms (or your favorite)
- 4 cups of low-sodium chicken or vegetable broth
- 1 (14.5 oz) can of diced tomatoes, undrained
- 1 bay leaf
- 1/2 tsp dried thyme
- 1/4 tsp dried oregano
- Pinch of saffron (optional)
- Salt and pepper to taste
- 12 oz. raw shrimp, peeled and deveined

Optional additions:

- 1 tbsp tomato paste
- Handful of chopped fresh parsley
- Cooked brown rice or quinoa

Instructions

1. Olive oil should be heated in a big pot or Dutch oven on medium heat.
2. Cook for 3-4 minutes until the chopped onions soften. Put some minced garlic and cook for an extra minute. It will become fragrant.
3. Slightly cook the chopped bell peppers and zucchini for approximately five to seven minutes.
4. Incorporate properly sliced mushrooms, then cook for 3-4 more minutes until it softens slightly.
5. Add the chicken or vegetable broth, diced tomatoes with their juices, bay leaf, herbs (thyme, oregano), and saffron (optional). Let it boil, then reduce the fire and simmer for about 10 minutes.
6. The soup should have enough salt and pepper to taste. Mix gently in peeled, deveined shrimp, then stir-fry until they turn pink within two to three minutes.
7. Alternatively, add tomato paste to make the soup thicker (optional). Serve hot, garnished with chopped parsley leaves (optional) over cooked brown rice or quinoa.

Nutrition per serving:

Calories: 300 Fat: 10g Carbs: 25g
Protein: 35g

Lentil & Kale Soup

Prep time: 15 minutes Cook time: 45 minutes Servings: 4-6

Ingredients

For the soup:

- 1 tbsp olive oil
- 1 onion, chopped
- 2 cloves garlic, minced
- 1 carrot, peeled and diced
- 1 celery stalk, diced
- 1 cup of green beans, trimmed and chopped
- 1 red bell pepper, diced
- 4 cups of low-sodium vegetable broth
- 1 (14.5 oz) can of diced tomatoes, undrained
- 1 cup of brown lentils, rinsed
- 1 bunch of kale, stems removed and leaves roughly chopped
- 1 bay leaf
- 1/2 tsp dried thyme
- 1/4 tsp dried rosemary
- Pinch of red pepper flakes (optional)
- Salt and pepper to taste

Optional additions:

- 1 tbsp tomato paste
- Handful of chopped fresh parsley
- Cooked brown rice or quinoa

Instructions

1. Heat the olive oil in a big saucepan or Dutch oven over medium heat.
2. When the onion is softened, add it and sauté it for three to four minutes. Add the minced garlic and stir until fragrant, about one more minutes.
3. Add the red bell pepper, green beans, celery, and chopped carrot. Simmer for 5 to 7 minutes or until somewhat tender.
4. Add the bay leaf, thyme, rosemary, chopped tomatoes with their juices, and optional red pepper flakes to the vegetable broth. After bringing it to a boil, lower the heat and simmer it for ten minutes.
5. Add the chopped kale and rinsed brown lentils. Let it simmer for 20 to 25 minutes or until the kale has wilted and the lentils are soft.
6. Add salt and pepper to taste when preparing the broth. For a thicker consistency, whisk in tomato paste if desired. If desired, serve hot cooked quinoa or brown rice and garnish with chopped fresh parsley.

Nutrition per serving:

Calories: 400 Fat: 15g Carbs: 35g Protein: 30g

Broccoli Soup

Prep time: 15 minutes Cook time: 25 minutes Servings: 4-6

Ingredients

For the soup:

- 1 tbsp olive oil
- 1 onion, chopped
- 2 cloves garlic, minced
- 1 head broccoli, florets chopped and stalks thinly sliced
- 4 cups of low-sodium vegetable broth
- 1/2 cup of unsweetened almond milk
- 1/4 cup of nutritional yeast
- 1/2 tsp dried thyme
- Pinch of nutmeg
- Salt and pepper to taste

Optional additions:

- 1 tbsp heavy cream or coconut cream
- Handful of chopped fresh parsley
- Crusty bread or crackers for dipping

Instructions

1. Heat the olive oil in a big saucepan or Dutch oven over medium heat.
2. When the onion is softened, add it and sauté it for three to four minutes. Add the minced garlic and stir until fragrant, about 1 more minute.
3. After adding the thinly sliced broccoli stalks, simmer for a further three to four minutes or until the stalks start to soften.
4. Stir in the almond milk (or milk), nutritional yeast (if using), nutmeg, thyme, and salt & pepper. After bringing it to a boil, lower the heat and simmer it for ten minutes.
5. Blend the soup until it's smooth and creamy by using an immersion blender or putting it in batches into a blender. If necessary, thin the mixture with more water or broth.
6. Add the chopped broccoli florets and boil for five to seven minutes or until the broccoli is crisp-tender.
7. For a deeper taste, stir with coconut or heavy cream (optional). Add some finely chopped fresh parsley as a garnish and serve warm with whole-wheat bread or crackers for the best match with the Galveston Diet.

Nutrition per serving:

Calories: 200 Fat: 10g Carbs: 20g Protein: 10g

Asparagus Soup

Prep time: 15 minutes Cook time: 25 minutes Servings: 4-6

Ingredients

For the soup:

- 1 tbsp olive oil
- 1 onion, chopped
- 2 cloves garlic, minced

- 1 lb. asparagus, tough ends trimmed and chopped into 1-inch pieces
- 4 cups of low-sodium vegetable broth
- 1 cup of unsweetened almond milk
- 1/4 cup of nutritional yeast
- 1/2 tsp dried tarragon
- Pinch of freshly grated nutmeg
- Salt and pepper to taste

Optional additions

- 1 tbsp lemon juice
- Handful of chopped fresh chives
- Sour cream or Greek yogurt dollop
- Crusty bread or crackers for dipping

Instructions

1. Heat olive oil in a large pot or Dutch oven over medium heat.
2. Chop onions and sauté them for 3-4 minutes until they become soft. Add minced garlic and cook for not less than one minute.
3. Chop the asparagus and cook it for 5-7 minutes. It should turn out bright green, slightly darker, and tender.
4. Add vegetable broth, almond milk (or regular milk), nutritional yeast (optional), tarragon, nutmeg, salt, and pepper to your taste. Bring to a boil and let it simmer for 10 minutes at reduced heat.
5. Using an immersion blender, transfer the soup to a blender in batches and blend until smooth. If you want a thicker soup, add broth or water.
6. Optional lemon juice made the soup brighter. Sprinkle with fresh chives when serving hot with sour cream or Greek yogurt (optional) and some crusty bread or crackers.

Nutrition per serving:

Calories: 200 Fat: 10g Carbs: 20g Protein: 10g

Chicken & Tomato Stew

Prep time: 15 minutes Cook time: 30 minutes Servings: 4-6

Ingredients

For the stew:

- 1 tbsp olive oil
- 1 onion, chopped
- 2 cloves garlic, minced
- 1 lb. boneless, skinless chicken thighs, cut into bite-sized pieces
- 1 bell pepper (any color), chopped
- 1 zucchini, diced
- 1 tsp dried oregano
- 1/2 tsp dried thyme
- 1/4 tsp smoked paprika (optional)
- Pinch of red pepper flakes (optional)
- 1 (14.5 oz) can of diced tomatoes, undrained
- 4 cups of low-sodium chicken or vegetable broth
- 1 cup of baby spinach or kale, roughly chopped
- Salt and pepper to taste

Optional additions:

- Handful of chopped fresh parsley or cilantro
- Cooked quinoa or brown rice (for side serving)

Instructions

1. You need a large pot or Dutch oven to heat olive oil over medium heat.
2. The onion is chopped, followed by sautéing for 3-4 minutes until it softens. Then, stir in the minced garlic and cook for another minute till fragrant.
3. Put in the chicken pieces and cook for 5-7 minutes or until lightly browned on all sides.
4. When slightly softened, add the chopped bell pepper, zucchini, oregano, thyme, smoked paprika (optional), and red pepper flakes (optional) to it. The mixture should be cooked for 3-4 minutes.
5. Add diced tomatoes with their juices and chicken (or vegetable) broth. Allow it to boil and then simmer on low fire for 15-20 minutes or until chicken is done.
6. Stir in baby spinach or kale and cook an additional minute till wilted.
7. Season with salt and pepper; garnish with chopped fresh parsley or cilantro (optional) before serving hot and served with cooked quinoa or brown rice (optional).

Nutrition per serving:

Calories: 350 Fat: 15g Carbs: 30g Protein: 35g

Chicken & Veggie Stew

Prep time: 15 minutes Cook time: 30 minutes Servings: 4-6

Ingredients

For the stew:

- 1 tbsp olive oil
- 1 onion, chopped
- 2 cloves garlic, minced
- 1 lb. boneless, skinless chicken thighs, cut into bite-sized pieces
- 1 bell pepper (any color), chopped
- 1 zucchini, diced
- 1 carrot, peeled and diced
- 1 celery stalk, diced
- 1 tsp dried oregano
- 1/2 tsp dried thyme
- Pinch of ground cumin
- Pinch of red pepper flakes (optional)
- 1 (14.5 oz) can of diced tomatoes, undrained
- 4 cups of low-sodium chicken or vegetable broth
- 1 cup of (cooked) quinoa or brown rice (per serving, optional)
- Salt and pepper to taste

Optional additions:

- Handful of chopped fresh parsley or cilantro
- Chopped avocado slices

- A dollop of plain Greek yogurt or coconut yogurt

Instructions

1. Olive oil should be heated in a large pot or Dutch oven over medium heat.
2. The chopped onion should be added and sautéed for 3-4 minutes until it becomes soft. After that, stir in the minced garlic and cook for another minute to bring out its aroma.
3. The chicken pieces should be added and cooked for 5-7 minutes until lightly browned on all sides.
4. Stir in the chopped bell pepper, zucchini, carrot, celery, oregano, thyme, cumin, and red pepper flakes (optional). Cook for an additional 5 minutes until they start to soften slightly.
5. Diced tomatoes with their juices and chicken or vegetable broth must be added. Bring to a boil, then reduce heat and simmer for 15-20 minutes or until chicken is cooked through.
6. Season the broth to taste with salt and pepper. Add some garnishing of chopped fresh parsley or cilantro (optional).
7. A scoop of cooked quinoa or brown rice per serving can be served hot (optional). Other options include sliced avocado, plain Greek yogurt, or coconut yogurt dollop.

Nutrition per serving:

Calories: 400 Fat: 15g Carbs: 30g
Protein: 35g

Beef & Tomato Stew

Prep time: 15 minutes Cook time: 1.5-2 hours Servings: 4-6

Ingredients

For the stew:

- 1 tbsp olive oil
- 1 onion, chopped
- 2 cloves garlic, minced
- 1 lb. boneless, chuck roast or stewing beef, cut into bite-sized pieces
- 1 bell pepper (any color), chopped
- 1 zucchini, diced
- 1 carrot, peeled and diced
- 1 celery stalk, diced
- 1 tsp dried oregano
- 1/2 tsp dried thyme
- Pinch of smoked paprika
- Pinch of red pepper flakes (optional)
- 1 (14.5 oz) can of diced tomatoes, undrained
- 4 cups of low-sodium beef or vegetable broth
- 1 cup of dry quinoa or brown rice (per serving, optional)
- Salt and pepper to taste

Optional additions:

- Handful of chopped fresh parsley or cilantro
- Chopped avocado slices
- A dollop of plain Greek yogurt or coconut yogurt

Instructions

1. Medium heat should be used to heat olive oil in a large pot or Dutch oven.
2. It will take three to four minutes of sautéing the chopped onion to become soft. After that, add the minced garlic and cook for an additional minute to make it smell nice.
3. You have to brown the beef pieces on all sides, which will take around five to seven minutes.
4. When tenderly cooked, add the chopped bell pepper, zucchini, carrot, celery, oregano, thyme, paprika, and red pepper flakes (optional). Cook for another 5 minutes until they become slightly soft.
5. Finally, add diced tomatoes with their juices and beef or vegetable broth. Bring to a boil; then reduce heat and simmer for 1½-2 hours until meat is tender and falling apart.
6. You can cook quinoa or brown rice according to package instructions while the stew simmers.
7. Salt and pepper should be added if you want a taste in your broth. For those who wish to garnish, use chopped fresh parsley or cilantro (optional).
8. Alternatively, serve hot with quinoa or brown rice per serving (optional). You may also consider serving it with avocado slices, plain Greek yogurt, or coconut yogurt.

Nutrition per serving:

Calories: 400 Fat: 20g Carbs: 35g
Protein: 40g

CHAPTER 4: MEAT RECIPES

Charcoal-Grilled Ribeye Steak

Prep time: 15 Cook time: 5-10 minutes Servings: 2

Ingredients

For the steak:

- 2 ribeye steaks (1-1.5 inches thick)
- 1 tbsp olive oil
- 1/2 tsp kosher salt
- 1/4 tsp freshly ground black pepper
- Optional: 1/2 tsp of your favorite steak seasoning

For the sides (optional):

- Grilled asparagus or zucchini
- Steamed broccoli or green beans
- Side salad with vinaigrette dressing
- Cooked quinoa or brown rice

Instructions

1. Bring the steaks to room temperature by taking them from the refrigerator for 30 minutes before cooking. Dry them with paper towels.
2. Rub olive oil all over the steaks. Salt, pepper, and your favorite steak seasoning can be added in generous amounts.
3. Prepare your charcoal grill for high direct heat (about 450°F to 500°F). Ensure that you have a uniform layer of hot coals.
4. Put the steaks on the hot grill and cook for 2-3 minutes per side or as desired. Your goal is to achieve a beautiful crust on the outside while keeping it moist inside.
5. Remove the steaks from the grill onto a plate, cover them loosely with foil, and let rest for about five or ten minutes before slicing. It is necessary that for a more tender and flavorful steak, juices be allowed to redistribute.

Nutrition per serving

Calories: 600 Fat: 35g Carbs: 0g Protein: 60g

Air Fryer New York Strip Steak

Prep time: 15 minutes Cook time: 12-16 minutes Servings: 2

Ingredients

For the steak:

- 2 New York strip steaks (1-1.5 inches thick)
- 1 tbsp olive oil
- 1/2 tsp kosher salt
- 1/4 tsp freshly ground black pepper
- Optional: 1/2 tsp of your favorite steak seasoning

For the sides (optional):

- Roasted broccoli or Brussels sprouts
- Steamed green beans or asparagus
- Side salad with vinaigrette dressing
- Cooked quinoa or brown rice

Instructions

1. The steaks should be brought to room temperature by removing them from the refrigerator 30 minutes before cooking. Dry them with a paper towel.
2. Coat the steaks with olive oil. You can also salt and pepper and add your favorite seasoning, such as steak.
3. Air fryers need preheating at 400°F (205°C) for 5 minutes.
4. Lay the steaks on the air fryer basket. The basket should not be overcrowded since this would affect the cooking temperature. For a medium rare, cook for about six to eight minutes per side or as per your taste for doneness.
5. Put the steaks on a plate and cover it tightly with foil for 5-10 minutes before slicing. Doing this ensures that tenderness and flavor are well mixed in a better steak by allowing juices to redistribute.

Nutrition per serving:

Calories: 500 Fat: 25g Carbs: 0g Protein: 50g

Instant Pot Corned Beef

Prep time: 15 minutes Cook time: 105 minutes Servings: 6-8

Ingredients

For the corned beef:

- 2-3 lb. corned beef brisket
- 4 cups of low-sodium vegetable broth
- 1 medium onion, roughly chopped (optional)
- 2-3 cloves garlic, smashed (optional)
- 1 bay leaf (optional)
- 1/2 tsp ground black pepper
- 1/4 tsp whole black peppercorns (optional)
- For the vegetables (optional):
- 2-3 carrots, peeled and chopped
- 2-3 potatoes, peeled and chopped
- 1 head cabbage, cored and quartered

For serving (optional):

- Whole-wheat bread or crackers
- Dijon mustard
- Horseradish sauce

Instructions

1. If your corned beef has a spice packet, wrap it in a cheesecloth bag or tin foil.
2. Pour vegetable broth into Instant Pot. Add chopped onion, garlic, bay leaf, ground pepper, and optional whole black peppercorns.
3. Drop the corned beef brisket fat side down into the Instant Pot liquid.

Place the spice packet on top of the meat if you're using it.

4. Secure the lid and set the pressure cooker on high for 90 minutes.
5. Allow 10 minutes for natural release, then manually release any remaining pressure.
6. Add carrots and potatoes to the Instant Pot when the corned beef rests and set on high pressure for 5 minutes. Quick release.
7. Add quartered cabbage and cook for 2-3 minutes until softened as desired.
8. Transfer carefully to the cutting board; let it sit for 10 minutes before carving against (across) its grain.
9. Serve with cooked vegetables (optional), whole-wheat bread/crackers, Dijon mustard, and horseradish sauce (optional).

Nutrition per serving

Calories: 300 Fat: 20g Carbs: 0g Protein: 35g

Slow Cooker Turkey Breast

Prep time: 15 minutes Cook time: 3-4 hours Servings: 4-6

Ingredients

For the turkey:

- 1 bone-in, skin-on turkey breast (4-5 lb.)
- 1 tbsp olive oil
- 1/2 tsp dried thyme
- 1/2 tsp dried sage
- 1/4 tsp salt
- 1/4 tsp black pepper
- 1 onion, roughly chopped (optional)
- 2 carrots, peeled and chopped (optional)
- 2 celery stalks, chopped (optional)
- 1 cup of low-sodium chicken or vegetable broth

For serving (optional):

- Brown rice or quinoa
- Steamed green beans or broccoli
- Cranberry sauce
- Whole-wheat rolls or stuffing

Instructions

1. Ensure your slow cooker is on low heat to preheat. Dab the breast of the turkey with a paper towel until it is dry. Brush it with olive oil and season thoroughly with thyme, sage, salt, and pepper.
2. If you have any, scatter the chopped onion, carrots, and celery in the bottom of the crockpot.
3. Put the seasoned turkey breast on top of the aromatics, if desired, by placing it sideways so that its breast side faces upwards. If you have any, pour broth at the base of the turkey.
4. Cover a slow cooking pot; hence, cook for 3-4 hours on low or until the internal temperature at the thickest part of a turkey breast reads 165°F.

5. Place turkey on the cutting board; let it remain for 10-15 minutes without carving.

6. Serve thinly sliced turkey with optional sides.

Nutrition per serving:

Calories: 250 Fat: 10g Carbs: 0g
Protein: 40g

Marinated Turkey Breast

Prep time: 15 minutes Cook time: 1-1.5 hours (roasting) or 45-60 minutes (grilling) Servings: 4-6

Ingredients

For the marinade:

- 1/4 cup of olive oil
- 2 tbsp fresh lemon juice
- 2 tbsp Dijon mustard
- 1 tbsp chopped fresh rosemary
- 1 tbsp chopped fresh thyme
- 1 tsp dried oregano
- 1/2 tsp garlic powder
- 1/4 tsp salt
- 1/4 tsp black pepper

For the turkey:

- 1 bone-in, skin-on turkey breast (4-5 lb.)
- For serving (optional):
- Brown rice or quinoa
- Steamed or roasted vegetables
- Grilled fruit or fresh salad

Instructions

1. Whisk the marinade ingredients in a mixing bowl or large zip-lock bag.

2. Make sure that the turkey breast is completely covered by it. Then, cover it and place it in the fridge for no less than four hours or longer if you desire more flavor.

3. Set your oven to 400°F (205°C) or heat the grill to medium-high temperature. Set up a baking rack with turkey breast over the roasting pan if you are roasting. In case of grilling, preheat your grill with oiled grates.

4. Roast turkey for about one and a half hours or 45-60 minutes on the grill, flipping once at mid-point. Additional marinade can be used while basting if required. The thickest part's internal temperature should be 165 degrees.

5. Then, transfer the turkey to a cutting board and let it rest for 10-15 minutes before slicing.

6. Slice thin servings of Turkey and accompany them with sides of choice (optional).

Nutrition per serving:

Calories: 300 Fat: 15g Carbs: 0g
Protein: 40g

Air Fryer Turkey Breast

Prep time: 15 minutes Cook time: 40-45 minutes Servings: 4-6

Ingredients

For the turkey:

- 1 bone-in, skin-on turkey breast (4-5 lb.)
- 1 tbsp olive oil
- 1/2 tsp dried thyme
- 1/2 tsp dried sage
- 1/4 tsp salt
- 1/4 tsp black pepper

For the sides (optional):

- Roasted Brussels sprouts or broccoli
- Steamed green beans or asparagus
- Side salad with vinaigrette dressing
- Brown rice or quinoa

Instructions

1. Switch on the air fryer and set it to 400°F (205°C) for under five minutes. Remove all moisture from the turkey breast using a paper towel. Then, use olive oil to brush it, and season it with thyme, sage, salt, and pepper.
2. On the other hand, if your air fryer's basket is large enough, you can put the turkey breast inside, side up, and tuck wing tips beneath it; otherwise, cut the breast into two halves to fit.
3. If you cook a four-pound breast, roast it for between forty and forty-five minutes or adjust the time according to size. Check the temperature in the thickest part of the turkey after thirty minutes; it should be above sixty-five for safety measures.
4. Place turkey on the carving board for ten to fifteen minutes before slicing. This way, juices will flow around, making birds taste better.
5. Thinly slice turkey and serve with accompanying sides as desired.

Nutrition per serving

Calories: 250 Fat: 10g Carbs: 0g Protein: 40g

Air Fryer Turkey Breast

Prep time: 15 minutes Cook time: 40-45 minutes Servings: 4-6

Ingredients

For the turkey:

- 1 bone-in, skin-on turkey breast (4-5 lb.)
- 1 tbsp olive oil
- 1/2 tsp dried thyme
- 1/2 tsp dried sage
- 1/4 tsp salt
- 1/4 tsp black pepper

For the sides (optional):

- Roasted Brussels sprouts or broccoli
- Steamed green beans or asparagus
- Side salad with vinaigrette dressing
- Brown rice or quinoa

Instructions

1. Pat the turkey breast dry with paper towels. Generously brush it with olive oil. Rub thyme, sage, salt, and pepper into the skin and flesh.
2. If you like, score the skin diagonally with a sharp knife to create crisscrossing patterns of shallow cuts about 1/4 inch deep. This will make the fat melt and the skin brown nicely.
3. Set your air fryer to preheat for 5 minutes at 400°F (205°C). For small air fryers, you may split the breast lengthwise.
4. Put the turkey breast in the air fryer basket with its skin side up. The basket should be manageable because it affects airflow and cooking time.
5. Cook for 40-45 minutes, depending on size if it is a 4-lb. breast. After 30 minutes, check for internal temperature in the thickest part of your breast meat. It should be 165°F to be safe for consumption.
6. Place turkey on a cutting board and let it stand for 10-15 minutes before slicing. This is done to distribute all juices evenly, making it a more tender and flavorful bird.
7. Thinly slice the turkey and serve it with your favorite sides (optional).

Nutrition per serving:

Calories: 250 Fat: 10g Carbs: 0g Protein: 40g

Roasted Rack of Lamb

Prep time: 10 minutes Cook time: 20-25 minutes Servings: 4-6

Ingredients

For the lamb:

- 2 racks of lamb (8-10 ribs each)
- 1 tbsp olive oil
- 1/2 tsp dried rosemary
- 1/2 tsp dried thyme
- 1/4 tsp salt
- 1/4 tsp black pepper

For the sides (optional):

- Roasted root vegetables (potatoes, carrots, parsnips)
- Steamed green beans or asparagus
- Quinoa or brown rice
- Fresh herb salad with vinaigrette dressing

Instructions

1. Preheat your oven to 425°F (220°C). Trim any excess fat from the lamb racks. Mix olive oil, rosemary, thyme, salt, and pepper in a small bowl. Massage the mixture over the lamb racks.
2. Arrange these racks of lamb on a roasting pan so that their fat side faces upwards. Add some water or broth at the bottom if you need it more moistened. Roast for about 20 to 25 minutes if you prefer medium rare, or adjust depending on how you want it done regarding doneness. Slice open with an instant-read thermometer to

ascertain internal temperature: generally speaking, medium rare is about 135°F while medium is around 145°F.

3. Cut into a board and let rest for ten minutes before slicing. Ten minutes of rest will allow for juicier meat with better taste.
4. Slice the lamb through the bones and serve with other sides if desired.

Nutrition per serving:

Calories: 400 Fat: 25g Carbs: 0g Protein: 40g

Roasted Lamb Breast

Prep time: 15 minutes Cook time: 2-2.5 hours Servings: 4-6

Ingredients

For the lamb:

- 1 bone-in lamb breast (4-5 lb.)
- 2 tbsp olive oil
- 1 tsp dried rosemary
- 1/2 tsp dried thyme
- 1/2 tsp garlic powder
- 1/4 tsp salt
- 1/4 tsp black pepper
- Optional: 1 onion, chopped (quartered) and one carrot, chopped (quartered) for roasting alongside

For serving (optional):

- Roasted or mashed potatoes
- Steamed green beans or broccoli
- Couscous or quinoa
- Fresh herb salad with vinaigrette dressing

Instructions

1. Your oven should be preheated to 325°F (163°C). The lamb breast should then be patted dry using paper towels. Mix olive oil, rosemary, thyme, garlic powder, salt, and pepper in a small bowl. Spread the mixture over the lamb breast to coat the meat and fat cap.
2. You can tie the lamb breast with kitchen twine at intervals to ensure it does not scatter while being cooked. It is unnecessary, but this can ensure that it does not break up as much during cooking.
3. Arrange the lamb breast in a roasting pan with the fat side facing up. Alternatively, spread chopped onions and carrots around the base of your pan if desired.
4. Put the pan into a preheated oven and roast for 2-2.5 hours or until the internal temperature of the thickest part of the meat reaches 165°F for safe consumption. You may prefer to baste your meat with juices every 30 minutes.
5. To carve a more succulent and flavorful result, leave it on the other end and let it sit for at least 15 minutes before cutting. Slice across grain thin lamb separating from bone meats.
6. Serve sliced lamb alongside preferred sides (optional). The roasted vegetables in the pan are

very delicious when served with them.

Nutrition per serving:

Calories: 350 Fat: 20g Carbs: 0g
Protein: 40g

Grilled Lamb Loin Chops

Prep time: 10 minutes Cook time: 6-8 minutes Servings: 4

Ingredients

For the lamb loin chops:

- 4 bone-in lamb loin chops (1-inch thick)
- 1 tbsp olive oil
- 1/2 tsp dried rosemary
- 1/2 tsp dried thyme
- 1/4 tsp garlic powder
- 1/4 tsp salt
- 1/4 tsp black pepper

For serving (optional):

- Grilled or roasted vegetables (asparagus, zucchini, bell peppers)
- Mashed or roasted potatoes
- Quinoa or brown rice
- Fresh herb salad with vinaigrette dressing

Instructions

1. Pat the lamb chops dry with a paper towel.
2. Put olive oil, rosemary, thyme, garlic powder, salt, and pepper in a small bowl. Mix them well. Spread this mixture generously over the chops so they are entirely coated inside and out.
3. Get ready for your grill by lighting it to medium-high heat. If you have a charcoal grill, you should wait until the coals turn medium-hot, which is a white ash color with some red embers.
4. Transfer the lamb chops onto the grill that has already been heated up. Cook 3-4 minutes per side to have medium-rare or as desired. For instance, if you prefer medium rare, let them cook for an extra 2 minutes on each side, and they will be done perfectly. To check if it's done, use an instant-read thermometer: in terms of the internal temperature, 135°F for Medium-Rare and 145°F for medium.
5. Remove from heat and keep aside for about ten minutes before serving. Redistribute juices to get succulent and flavorful results.
6. Place your preferred garnish (optional) and grilled lamb loin chops on your plate. Grilled lamb goes nicely with herb salad, fresh veggies, and tables, though the sides can accompany it.

Nutrition per serving:

Calories: 350 Fat: 20g Carbs: 0g
Protein: 40g

Weeknight Skillet Slaw

Prep time: 15 minutes Cook time: 10-12 minutes Servings: 4

Ingredients

For the slaw:

- 4 cups of thinly sliced green cabbage
- 1 cup of shredded carrots
- 1/2 cup of chopped red onion
- 1/4 cup of chopped fresh parsley

For the chicken:

- 1 lb. boneless, skinless chicken breasts or thighs, thinly sliced
- 1 tbsp olive oil
- 1/2 tsp salt
- 1/4 tsp black pepper

For the dressing:

- 2 tbsp apple cider vinegar
- 1 tbsp olive oil
- 1 tsp Dijon mustard
- 1/2 tsp honey
- 1/4 tsp salt
- 1/4 tsp black pepper
- For serving (optional):
- Brown rice or quinoa
- Whole-wheat tortillas or wraps
- Fresh avocado slices
- Chopped fresh herbs like cilantro or mint

Instructions

1. Mix shredded cabbage, carrots, red onion, and parsley in a large bowl. Keep aside.

2. In a large skillet, heat olive oil over medium-high heat. Sprinkle the chicken slices with salt and pepper, add to the skillet, and cook for four to five minutes until golden brown and cooked through.

3. While the chicken is cooking, whisk all dressing ingredients together in a small bowl or jar until emulsified.

4. Once the chicken is done cooking, place it on a plate. Mix well with the slaw mixture with the dressing.

5. Plate the slaw mixture and top with cooked chicken slices or other optional toppings.

6. The above-finished recipe provides portions suitable for approximately four servings.

Nutrition per serving:

Calories: 400 Fat: 20g Carbs: 20g Protein: 35g

Easy Pork Tenderloin

Prep time: 10 minutes Cook time: 20-25 minutes Servings: 4-6

Ingredients:

For the tenderloin:

- 1 pork tenderloin (1-1.5 lb.)
- 1 tbsp olive oil
- 1/2 tsp dried thyme
- 1/2 tsp dried rosemary
- 1/4 tsp garlic powder
- 1/4 tsp salt
- 1/4 tsp black pepper

For serving (optional):

- Roasted vegetables
- Steamed green beans or asparagus
- Quinoa or brown rice
- Fresh herb salad with vinaigrette dressing

Instructions

1. Preheat your oven to 400°F (205°C). Trim any surplus fat from the pork tenderloin. Mix olive oil, thyme, rosemary, garlic powder, salt, and pepper in a small bowl. Generously apply this combination to the tenderloin, ensuring it is used on both sides.
2. Heat a large skillet over medium-high heat with a drizzle of olive oil for extra flavor and browning. Brown the tenderloin for 2-3 minutes per side until golden brown. It's just a nice thing to add but optional.
3. Transfer the seasoned tenderloin to a roasting pan or baking sheet. If you were searing, add some splash of water or broth into the pan to avoid dryness. Roast for 20-25 minutes until internal temperature reaches 145°F for safe consumption. To get it right, use your meat thermometer here.
4. Once baked, remove the tenderloin from the oven and let it stand for ten minutes before carving. This will make it taste more delicious and yielding due to the even distribution of juices. Thinly slice the tenderloin against the grain.
5. Plate with optional sides after slicing pork into thin slices. Also, fresh herbs like parsley or thyme can be added as a finishing touch.

Nutrition per serving:

Calories: 250 Fat: 10g Carbs: 0g
Protein: 40g

Chicken Lettuce Wraps

Prep time: 10 minutes Cook time: 20 minutes Servings: 4-6

Ingredients

For the filling:

- 1 lb. ground chicken (90% lean or higher)
- 1 tbsp sesame oil
- 1/2 cup of chopped onion
- 2 cloves garlic, minced
- 1 inch fresh ginger, grated
- 1 red bell pepper, diced
- 1/2 cup of water chestnuts, diced (optional)
- 1/4 cup of soy sauce
- 1 tbsp rice vinegar
- 1 tsp brown sugar
- 1/2 tsp sriracha
- 1/4 tsp black pepper
- 1/4 cup of chopped fresh cilantro

For serving:

- 12 large butter lettuce leaves, washed and dried
- Optional toppings: chopped peanuts, sliced avocado, shredded carrots, cucumber sticks, hoisin sauce

Instructions

1. Heat the sesame oil in a large skillet over medium-high heat. While you are browning it, break the ground chicken up with a spoon.
2. Add onion, garlic, and ginger to the pan and cook until softened, about 1-2 minutes. Additionally, bell pepper and water chestnuts cook for another 2-3 minutes.
3. Whisk together soy sauce, rice vinegar, brown sugar (if using), Sriracha, and black pepper; pour into the skillet and simmer. Finally, thicken slightly over 2-3 minutes of cooking.
4. Remove from heat, then stir in the cilantro that you have chopped. Meanwhile, put some chicken filling on each leaf of lettuce and lay other toppings upon them.

Nutrition per serving:

Calories: 300 Fat: 15g Carbs: 15g Protein: 35g

Easy Air Fryer Whole Chicken

Prep time: 10 minutes Cook time: 50-60 minutes Servings: 4-6

Ingredients:

- 1 whole chicken (3-4 lb.)
- 1 tbsp olive oil
- 1/2 tsp dried thyme
- 1/2 tsp dried rosemary

- 1/4 tsp garlic powder
- 1/4 tsp salt
- 1/4 tsp black pepper

Instructions:

1. Use paper towels to pat the chicken dry, including the cavity, and remove any giblets.
2. Mix olive oil, thyme, rosemary, garlic powder, salt, and pepper in a small bowl. Rub this mixture generously over the chicken to ensure its skin and cavity are well coated.
3. Preheat your air fryer to 375°F (190°C). Get the air fryer hot before cooking anything in it.
4. Carefully put the chicken breast-side down in the air fryer basket. If you have a small basket, you may need to tuck your wings under its body.
5. Cook for 30 minutes, flip the chicken, and cook for an additional 20-30 minutes, or until internal temperature at the thickest part of the thigh has reached 165°F for safety.
6. Take the chicken out of the air fryer and rest for 10-15 minutes before carving. This helps distribute juices, making for a more tender and flavorful outcome. Carve the chicken into serving pieces, and enjoy!

Nutrition per serving:

Calories: 350 Fat: 20g Carbs: 0g
Protein: 40g

Lemon-Roasted Chicken

Prep time: 15 minutes Cook time: 1 hour 15 minutes Servings: 4-6

Ingredients

For the chicken:

- 1 whole chicken (3-4 lb.)
- 1 lemon, halved
- 2 tbsp olive oil
- 1 tsp dried thyme
- 1/2 tsp dried rosemary
- 1/2 tsp garlic powder
- 1/4 tsp salt
- 1/4 tsp black pepper

For serving (optional):

- Roasted vegetables
- Steamed green beans or asparagus
- Quinoa or brown rice
- Fresh herb salad with vinaigrette dressing

Instructions

1. The oven should be preheated to 425°F (220°C). Use a paper towel to dry the chicken, including inside the cavity. Remove giblets if they are included.
2. Mix olive oil, thyme, rosemary, garlic powder, salt, and pepper in a small bowl. Rub all over the chicken, ensuring it is well coated on the skin and the cavity.
3. Put half of the lemon into the chicken's body cavity and the other half on its breast skin.
4. Place your chicken in a roasting pan with its breasts facing upwards.

Roast for about 1 hour and 15 minutes or until an internal temperature of 165°F in the thickest part of the thigh is reached. Baste pan juices over your chicken every 20-30 minutes for extra flavor and moistness.

5. After removing it from the oven, let it rest for ten to fifteen minutes before the car because it helps redistribute juices, resulting in more tenderness and flavor. Serve by carving the meat into pieces!

Nutrition per serving:

Calories: 400 Fat: 20g Carbs: 0g
Protein: 45g

Boiled Chicken

Prep time: 10 minutes Cook time: 20-45 minutes

Ingredients

- 1 whole chicken
- Water

Optional:

- 1-2 carrots, chopped
- 1-2 onions, quartered
- 1 celery stalk, chopped
- 1 bay leaf
- 1 tsp dried thyme
- 1/2 tsp black peppercorns

Instructions

1. A large pot should be used to put the whole chicken or desired chicken parts. If it is a whole chicken, take away any giblets.
2. Ensure the chicken is completely submerged in cold water by at least one inch.
3. Additionally, one can include chopped vegetables, bay leaf, thyme, and peppercorns in the pot to give the chicken more flavor.
4. Let it come to a boil over medium-high heat. During this time, remove any foam on top of the water.
5. Once boiling has started, reduce heat to low so you can simmer for 20-25 minutes for boneless skinless chicken breasts or thighs or 40-45 minutes for a whole bird. This depends on the size as well as the thickness of the pieces.
6. It is necessary to use a meat thermometer after following the recommended cooking time to check the internal temperature at its thickest part, which should be at least 165°F for consumption safety.
7. While still hot, transfer cooked chicken onto a plate and leave until cool enough so that you can shred using two forks if preferred.
8. Bored chicken can be used in your favorite recipes, salads, or sliced with dipping sauce as a light and healthy snack.

Nutrition per serving

Calories: 165 Fat: 3g Carbs: 0g
Protein: 35g

<u>Simple Lemon Herb Chicken</u>

Prep time: 10 minutes Cook time: 20-25 minutes Servings: 4

Ingredients

For the chicken:

- 4 boneless, skinless chicken breasts
- 1 tbsp olive oil
- 1/2 tsp dried thyme
- 1/2 tsp dried rosemary
- 1/4 tsp garlic powder
- 1/4 tsp salt
- 1/4 tsp black pepper
- 1/2 lemon, juiced

For serving (optional):

- Roasted vegetables
- Steamed green beans or asparagus
- Quinoa or brown rice
- Fresh herb salad with vinaigrette dressing

Instructions

1. Preheat your oven to 400°F (205°C). Use parchment paper to line a baking sheet.
2. Whisk olive oil, thyme, rosemary, garlic powder, salt, pepper, and lemon juice in a small bowl.
3. Put the chicken breasts in a shallow dish and pour marinade over them. Mix well.
4. Place the coated chicken on the prepared baking sheet and bake for 20-25 minutes or until done and brownish-golden in color.
5. Serve the roasted chicken with your preferred sides and taste the sunshine!
6. Heat olive oil in a large skillet over medium-high heat.
7. Mix herbs and spices to season chicken breast. Sear for 3-4 minutes per side until golden brown and cooked through.
8. Pour lemon juice into the pan and deglaze (scrape up any browned bits) for 30 seconds to give the chicken extra lemon flavor.
9. Place seared chicken on a plate along with pan drippings; enjoy the crispy finish with your favorite sides.

Nutrition per serving

Calories: 300 Fat: 15g Carbs: 0g
Protein: 40g

<u>Thai Ginger Chicken</u>

Prep time: 15 minutes Cook time: 10-15 minutes Servings: 4

Ingredients

For the chicken:

- 1 lb. boneless, skinless chicken breasts or thighs, thinly sliced
- 1 tbsp cornstarch
- 1/2 tsp salt
- 1/4 tsp black pepper

For the sauce:

- 2 tbsp coconut oil

- 2 tbsp light soy sauce (reduced sodium preferred)
- 1 tbsp brown sugar
- 1 tbsp rice vinegar
- 1 inch fresh ginger, grated
- 2 cloves garlic, minced
- 1 red chili pepper, thinly sliced (adjust to your spice preference)
- 1/2 cup of chicken broth
- 1/4 cup of fresh lime juice
- 1 tbsp chopped fresh cilantro

For serving (optional):

- Steamed white or brown rice
- Sauteed vegetables (broccoli, bell peppers, carrots)
- Fresh lime wedges for garnish

Instructions

1. Mix the chicken slices in a bowl with cornstarch, salt, and pepper, then let it marinate for 15 minutes.
2. Heat coconut oil in a large skillet or wok over medium-high heat.
3. Cook the chicken: Marinated chicken is put in and cooked for approximately 3-4 minutes on each side until golden brown and well done.
4. While the chicken cooks, blend soy sauce, brown sugar, rice vinegar, ginger garlic, and chili pepper in a small bowl.
5. Then, pour the sauce into the pan with the chicken and bring to a simmer once it's cooked. The sauce should be slightly thickened by boiling for 2-3 minutes.
6. Add lime juice and fresh cilantro; turn off the stove. Remove from heat and stir in lime juice and fresh cilantro. Eventually, remove the heat; stir in lime juice and fresh cilantro.
7. Serve Thai Ginger Chicken over rice with sautéed vegetables if desired, and garnish with fresh lime wedges to add citrusy sunshine to this dish.

Nutrition:

Calories: 400 Fat: 20g Carbs: 30g Protein: 35g

Juicy Grilled Chicken Breasts

Prep time: 10 minutes Cook time: 10-12 minutes Servings: 4

Ingredients

- 4 boneless, skinless chicken breasts
- 2 tbsp olive oil
- 1/2 tsp dried thyme
- 1/2 tsp dried rosemary
- 1/4 tsp garlic powder
- 1/4 tsp salt
- 1/4 tsp black pepper

Instructions

1. Pat the chicken breasts dry with paper towels, but if you like, you can slightly flatten them using a meat mallet for uniform thickness. If desired, it is possible to lb. them

lightly and evenly using a meat hammer.

2. Mix oil, thyme, rosemary, garlic powder, salt, and pepper in a small bowl to make the marinade. Pour this marinade over the chicken breast or brush it on.

3. Heat your grill to medium-high (nice and hot) for direct grilling, or use a grill pan on the stovetop if you don't have access to one.

4. Place marinated chicken breasts onto a preheated grill and cook for 4-5 minutes per side until thoroughly cooked and browned. You can test it with a meat thermometer that measures internal temperature at 165 degrees Fahrenheit, which is safe to consume.

5. Take off the grill and let sit for five to ten minutes before cutting or serving whole; this way, juices get distributed for more flavor and tenderness. This allows the juices in the meat to be redistributed so that they will be allocated for better taste and quality.

Nutrition per serving

Calories: 300 Fat: 15g Carbs: 0g Protein: 35-40g

Easy Chicken Cacciatore

Prep time: 15 minutes Cook time: 20-25 minutes Servings: 4

Ingredients

For the chicken:

- 4 boneless, skinless chicken breasts or thighs
- 1 tbsp olive oil
- 1/2 tsp salt
- 1/4 tsp black pepper

For the sauce:

- 1 tbsp olive oil
- 1/2 onion, chopped
- 1 green bell pepper, chopped
- 2 cloves garlic, minced
- 1 (28-oz.) can crushed tomatoes
- 1/2 cup of chicken broth
- 1 tsp dried oregano
- 1/2 tsp dried thyme
- Pinch of red pepper flakes (optional)
- 1/4 cup of fresh parsley, chopped (optional)

For serving (optional):

- Whole-wheat pasta or brown rice
- Sauteed green beans or spinach
- Crusty bread for dipping

Instructions

1. Start by preheating your oven at 400°F (205°C).

2. Pat dry the chicken, then season it with salt and pepper. Using medium-high heat, heat olive oil in

a large oven-proof skillet. Brown the chicken for 2-3 minutes on each side.

3. To the pan, add chopped onion, bell pepper, and garlic; cook for 3-4 minutes until soft. Crushed tomatoes, chicken broth, oregano, thyme, and red pepper flakes (if using); bring to a simmer, then scrape up any browned bits from the bottom of the pan.

4. Place chicken pieces in sauce; they should continue to simmer. Put a lid over the pan and bake for 20 to 25 minutes or until the chicken is done and the sauce has thickened somewhat.

5. You may sprinkle fresh parsley on top (optional) and serve with sides of your choice.

Nutrition:

Calories: 400 Fat: 20g Carbs: 30g Protein: 35g

Garlic Roasted Duck Breast

Prep time: 15 minutes Cook time: 25-30 minutes Servings: 2

Ingredients

- 2 duck breasts, skin on
- 2 tbsp olive oil
- 1 tsp dried thyme
- 1/2 tsp dried rosemary
- 1/4 tsp salt
- 1/4 tsp black pepper
- 4 cloves garlic, smashed

Instructions

1. Preheat oven to 400°F (200°C).
2. Skin side up, place the duck breasts on a cutting board. From there, score the skin using an extremely sharp knife in a diamond pattern, ensuring that one doesn't cut through to the meat.
3. Mix olive oil with thyme, rosemary, salt, and pepper in a small bowl. This should be rubbed on top of the duck breasts to cover the skin.
4. Place duck breasts on a roasting pan with skin side up. Spread crushed garlic cloves around the pan.
5. Roast for 20-25 minutes until the duck is fully cooked and has crispy skin. The internal temperature of the duck should reach 165°F (74°C).
6. Let them rest for five to ten minutes before slicing and serving them.

Nutrition per serving

Calories: 450 Protein: 35 g Fat: 35 g Carbohydrates: 3 g

Firecracker Salmon

Prep time: 10 minutes Cook time: 15-20 minutes Servings: 2

Ingredients

For the salmon:

- 2 salmon fillets (6-8 oz each)
- 1 tbsp soy sauce
- 1 tbsp honey or brown sugar
- 1 tbsp Sriracha sauce
- 1 tbsp grated ginger
- 1 tsp lime juice
- 1/2 tsp garlic powder
- 1/4 tsp black pepper
- Pinch of red pepper flakes (optional)

For serving (optional):

- Steamed brown rice or quinoa
- Roasted vegetables (broccoli, asparagus, bell peppers)
- Fresh lime wedges and chopped cilantro for garnish

Instructions

1. Start warming your oven to a temperature of 400°F (205°C)—lay parchment paper over a baking sheet.
2. In a small bowl, mix soy sauce, honey or brown sugar, Sriracha, ginger, lime juice, garlic powder, black pepper, and red pepper flakes (if you like). Put the marinated salmon fillets inside and turn them over to ensure they are evenly coated.
3. When done with marinating salmon, transfer it to the ready baking sheet and bake for about 15 -20 minutes or until fully cooked and the internal temperature is 145°F
4. Decorate Firecracker Salmon with preferred side dishes; drizzle some marinade sauce on top for an added touch. For an appealing finishing touch, include sliced fresh limes and cilantro.

Nutrition per serving:

Calories: 400 Fat: 20g Carbs: 30g Protein: 35g

Lemon-Pepper Salmon

Prep time: 10 minutes Cook time: 15-20 minutes Servings: 2

Ingredients

For the salmon:

- 2 salmon fillets
- 1 tbsp olive oil
- 1/2 tsp dried dill (optional)
- 1/2 tsp salt
- 1/4 tsp black pepper
- Zest of 1 lemon
- Freshly ground black pepper to taste

For serving (optional):

* Roasted vegetables
* Steamed brown rice or quinoa
* Fresh lemon wedges and chopped parsley for garnish

Instructions

1. Preheat your oven to 400 degrees Fahrenheit (205 degrees Celsius), then cover a baking pan with parchment paper.
2. Make sure you dry the fillets with paper towels. Use olive oil to brush them on both sides and sprinkle dill, salt, black pepper, and zest of lemon if using it.
3. Roast the fish for around 15 to 20 minutes, or until they are entirely cooked and their temperature reaches 145 degrees Fahrenheit internally.
4. Drizzle the pan juices over the Lemon-Pepper Salmon Plate with your preferred accompaniments to add flavor. For a fresh touch, garnish it with chopped lemon wedges and parsley.

Nutrition per serving

Calories: 300 Fat: 10-15g Carbs: 10g Protein: 35g

Spicy Garlic Salmon

Prep time: 10 minutes Cook time: 15-20 minutes Servings: 2

Ingredients:

For the salmon:

* 2 salmon fillets (6-8 oz each)
* 1 tbsp olive oil
* 1/2 tsp dried oregano
* 1/2 tsp smoked paprika (optional)
* 1/4 tsp salt
* 1/4 tsp black pepper
* 2 cloves garlic, minced
* 1/2 tsp red pepper flakes
* 1 tbsp Sriracha sauce (optional)

For serving (optional):

* Roasted vegetables (sweet potato, broccoli, peppers)
* Quinoa or brown rice pilaf
* Freshly chopped cilantro and lime wedges for garnish

Instructions

1. Preheat your oven to 400°F. Line a baking sheet with parchment paper.
2. Olive oil, oregano, paprika (if used), garlic, salt, pepper, red pepper flakes, and Sriracha (if used) should all be mixed in a small bowl. Salmon fillets should be equally brushed on both sides of the mixture.
3. After putting the salmon on the prepared baking sheet, roast it for 15 to 20 minutes or until the internal temperature reaches 145°F and is cooked.
4. Arrange the sides you've selected for the Spicy Garlic Salmon and pour over any pan juices for a flavor boost. For a vibrant final touch, garnish with lime wedges and chopped cilantro.

Nutrition per serving

Calories: 400 Fat: 20g Carbs: 25g Protein: 35g

Baked Dijon Salmon

Prep time: 10 minutes Cook time: 15-20 minutes Servings: 2

Ingredients:

For the salmon:

- 2 salmon fillets
- 1 tbsp olive oil
- 1/2 tsp dried thyme
- 1/4 tsp salt
- 1/4 tsp black pepper
- 2 tbsp Dijon mustard
- 1 tbsp honey or maple syrup

For serving (optional):

- Roasted vegetables (asparagus, Brussels sprouts, potatoes)
- Quinoa or brown rice pilaf
- Fresh lemon wedges and chopped parsley for garnish

Instructions

1. Preheat your oven to 400°F (205°C). Line a baking sheet with parchment paper.
2. Whisk together olive oil, thyme, salt, pepper, Dijon mustard, honey, or maple syrup in a small bowl. Ensure you brush the mixture steadily over the salmon fillets on both sides.
3. Place salmon fillets on prepared baking sheets and roast them for 15-20 minutes or until done and the internal temperature reaches 145°F.
4. Serve Baked Dijon Salmon on your selected accompaniments with some pan juices drizzled on top. Lastly, garnish with fresh lemon wedges and chopped parsley to add brightness.

Nutrition per serving

Calories: 400 Fat: 20g Carbs: 25g Protein: 35g

Pan-Seared Salmon

Prep time: 5 minutes Cook time: 10-12 minutes Servings: 2

Ingredients

For the salmon:

- 2 salmon fillets
- 1 tbsp olive oil
- 1/2 tsp of your chosen herb and spice blend

Herb and Spice Blend Options:

- 1/2 tsp dried dill, 1/4 tsp lemon zest, salt, pepper
- 1/2 tsp smoked paprika
- 1/4 tsp garlic powder
- pinch of cayenne pepper (optional), salt, pepper
- Steamed vegetables
- Quinoa or brown rice pilaf

* Fresh lemon wedges and chopped herbs for garnish

Instructions

1. To ensure a crispy sear, removing any moisture on the surface of fish fillets using paper towels is beneficial.
2. Take your chosen blend of herb and spice mix and olive oil. Pour this mixture equally all over both sides of salmon fillets.
3. Pan should be hot before adding the salmon to the skillet.
4. Cook salmon fillets for 3-4 minutes on each side or until golden brown and cooked through. The internal temperature should reach 145°F for safe consumption.
5. After cooking, let the salmon rest for about 5 minutes before transferring it to a plate. This allows the juices to be redistributed, thus maximizing flavor and tenderness.
6. This dish can be served with fresh lemon juice (optional) and some of your favorite side dishes. For added freshness, garnish with chopped herbs.

Nutrition per serving:

Calories: 400 Fat: 20g Carbs: 10g Protein: 35g

Lemon Rosemary Salmon

Prep time: 10 minutes Cook time: 15-20 minutes Servings: 2

Ingredients:

For the salmon:

* 2 salmon fillets
* 1 tbsp olive oil
* 1/2 tsp salt
* 1/4 tsp black pepper
* 2 sprigs fresh rosemary, plus additional for garnish
* Zest and juice of 1/2 lemon

For serving (optional):

* Roasted vegetables (zucchini, cherry tomatoes, bell peppers)
* Quinoa or brown rice pilaf
* Fresh lemon wedges and chopped parsley for garnish

Instructions

1. Preheat your oven to 400°F. Line a baking sheet with parchment paper.
2. Put the salmon fillets on the prepared baking sheet. Then, put some olive oil on top, along with salt, pepper, and lemon zest. Add a rosemary sprig beneath each fillet and pour lemon juice over it.
3. Bake for 15-20 minutes until it's done inside, and the internal thermometer reveals 145°F.
4. To serve, plate the Lemon Rosemary Salmon with your selected sides. Add extra remaining

rosemary sprigs and chopped parsley to garnish it.

Nutrition per serving:

Calories: 400 Fat: 20g Carbs: 10g Protein: 35g

Baked Asian Rockfish

Prep time: 15 minutes Cook time: 15-20 minutes Servings: 2

Ingredients

For the rockfish:

- 2 rockfish fillets (6-8 oz each)
- 1 tbsp soy sauce
- 1 tbsp toasted sesame oil
- 1 tbsp rice vinegar
- 1 tsp honey or brown sugar
- 1 tbsp grated ginger
- 1 clove garlic, minced
- 1/2 tsp toasted sesame seeds
- Pinch of red pepper flakes (optional)

For serving (optional):

- Steamed bok choy or broccoli
- Brown rice or quinoa pilaf
- Fresh scallions and chopped cilantro for garnish

Instructions

1. Preheat your oven to 400 degrees Fahrenheit. Use parchment paper to line a baking sheet.
2. In a small bowl, beat together soy sauce, vegetable oil, vinegar, honey/brown sugar, ginger, garlic, and the flakes of red pepper (optional). Placed in the marinade rockfish filets and coat the two sides uniformly. Allow it to sit for at least fifteen minutes or up to half an hour for more intense flavor.
3. Then, place the marinated rockfish on the prepared baking sheet. Drizzle them with any remaining marinade, then bake them for 15-20 minutes until fully cooked and the internal temperature registers 145°F. Halfway through, you should baste with remaining marine to improve flavor and moistness.
4. Plate Baked Asian Rockfish along with your preferred accompaniments. Sprinkle with toasted sesame seeds and chopped cilantro for visual effect and variety of experience.

Nutrition per serving:

Calories: 300 Fat: 15g Carbs: 25g Protein: 30g

Baked Asian Rockfish

Prep time: 15 minutes Cook time: 15-20 minutes Servings: 2

Ingredients:

For the rockfish:

- 2 rockfish fillets
- 1 tbsp soy sauce
- 1 tbsp toasted sesame oil
- 1 tbsp rice vinegar

- 1 tsp honey or brown sugar
- 1 tbsp grated ginger
- 1 clove garlic, minced
- 1/2 tsp toasted sesame seeds
- Pinch of red pepper flakes (optional)

For serving (optional):

- Steamed bok choy or broccoli
- Brown rice or quinoa pilaf
- Fresh scallions and chopped cilantro for garnish

Instructions

1. Preheat your oven to 400°F. Line a baking sheet with parchment paper.
2. Mix the rice vinegar, honey or brown sugar, ginger, garlic, red pepper flakes (if using), soy sauce, sesame oil, and rice vinegar in a small bowl. Coat the rockfish fillets equally on both sides by placing them in the marinade. If you want a deeper taste, marinate for up to 30 minutes, but at least 15 minutes is enough.
3. Once the baking sheet is ready, move the marinated rockfish to it. Brush with any leftover marinade and bake for 15 to 20 minutes or until cooked. A thermometer inserted in the center registers 145°F. Halfway through baking, baste the fish with the marinade to increase moisture and flavor.
4. Arrange the sides you want to go with the Baked Asian Rockfish. Toss in some chopped cilantro and

toasted sesame seeds for flavor and texture.

Nutrition per serving:

Calories: 300 Fat: 10g Carbs: 25g Protein: 35g

Thai Shrimp Wonton Cups

Prep time: 15 minutes Cook time: 25 minutes Servings: 24

Ingredients

For the wonton cups of:

- 24 wonton wrappers
- 1 ½ tbsp olive oil

For the filling:

- 1 tbsp olive oil
- 1 clove garlic, minced
- 1 tsp grated fresh ginger
- 8 oz. frozen medium shrimp, thawed, shelled, and deveined
- ½ lime, juiced
- 7 ½ oz. chive-and-onion cream cheese spread
- ¼ cup of Thai sweet chili sauce
- 1 green onion, chopped

For serving (optional):

- Fresh lime wedges
- Chopped cilantro

Instructions

1. Make your oven's preheating process to a temperature of 180°C (350°F). Lightly cover 24 cups of

mini muffin tins with cooking spray.

2. Lightly push a wonton wrapper into each muffin cup. Add olive oil on top. Cook for ten minutes until they become golden and crispy. Remove from the oven and allow cooling in the pans.

3. Warm olive oil in a large frying pan over medium heat. Put ginger and garlic inside, and cook for 30 seconds or until fragrant.

4. Insert shrimp, then cook them on either side for about three to four minutes per side until they turn pinkish and are properly cooked through. Then, you can just squeeze in some lime juice and mix well.

5. Blend cream cheese spread with Thai sweet chili sauce in a small bowl. Pour this mixture onto the cooked shrimp and stir it properly.

6. At that point, when wonton cups are cold enough, spoon shrimp mixture into each, then sprinkle green onions on top. Garnished with fresh wedges of lime and chopped cilantro would do better for an extra zest.

Nutrition per serving

Calories: 90 Fat: 5g Carbs: 10g Protein: 5g

Air Fryer Tilapia

Prep time: 5 minutes Cook time: 8-10 minutes Servings: 2

Ingredients

For the Tilapia:

- 2 Tilapia fillets (6-8 oz each)
- 1 tbsp olive oil
- 1/2 tsp paprika
- 1/4 tsp garlic powder
- 1/4 tsp salt
- 1/4 tsp black pepper
- Optional: Squeeze of lemon juice, your favorite herbs and spices

For Serving (Optional):

- Roasted vegetables (broccoli, asparagus, zucchini)
- Quinoa or brown rice pilaf
- Fresh lemon wedges and chopped parsley for garnish

Instructions

1. Then, wipe the fish fillets with paper towels and remove any excess moisture. This will help give it a crunchy texture.

2. Mix olive oil, paprika, garlic powder, salt, and pepper in another small bowl. Rub the mixture on all sides of the Tilapia fillets evenly. Or, if you want to have the added taste, consider squeezing some lemon juice or using your favorite herbs and spices.

3. Preheat your air fryer up to 400°F (205°C). Next, arrange seasoned Tilapia fillets in a single layer in the

air fryer basket. It takes about 8-10 minutes for them to be fully cooked and golden brown. For uniform browning, flip halfway through the cooking process.

4. Put the Air Fryer Tilapia on plates and with whatever else you need as an addition. Add fresh lemon wedges and finely chopped parsley to give the dish some color and zest.

5. Serve crispy tilapia with light yogurt sauce or your favorite dipping sauce for extra flavor and moistness.

Nutrition per serving:

Calories: 350 Fat: 20g Carbs: 10g
Protein: 30g

Pan-Seared Tilapia

Prep time: 5 minutes Cook time: 8-10 minutes Servings: 2

Ingredients

For the Tilapia:

- 2 Tilapia fillets (6-8 oz each)
- 1 tbsp olive oil
- 1/2 tsp paprika
- 1/4 tsp garlic powder
- 1/4 tsp salt
- 1/4 tsp black pepper

Optional: Squeeze of lemon juice, pinch of cayenne pepper

For Serving (Optional):

- Roasted vegetables (broccoli, asparagus, zucchini)
- Quinoa or brown rice pilaf
- Fresh lemon wedges and chopped parsley for garnish

Instructions:

1. Make sure you remove excess moisture by using paper towels to pat the fish fillets dry. This will ensure the fish has a crispy skin.

2. Mix olive oil, paprika, garlic powder, salt, and pepper in a small bowl. Spread the mixture evenly onto both sides of the Tilapia fillets. Add a pinch of cayenne or squeeze some lemon on top for that extra tang if desired.

3. Put a large non-stick skillet over medium-high heat. Once the pan gets hot enough with shimmering oil, put in the Tilapia fillets, but do not overcrowd.

4. Cook the fish for about 3-4 minutes per side until golden brown and cooked through. To make it safe for consumption, its internal temperature should be 145°F.

5. Take off heat once it is done; set it on a plate for about 5 minutes before serving. This allows the meat fibers to relax and take up fluids, moistening their flavor.

6. Just pick your favorite balanced diet and serve your pan-eared tilapia. On top of that, garnish with fresh lemon wedges and sprinkle chopped parsley to give it more style.

Nutrition per serving:

Calories: 300 Fat: 15g Carbs: 5g
Protein: 30g

Easy Baked Tilapia

Prep time: 5 minutes Cook time: 15-20 minutes Servings: 2

Ingredients

For the Tilapia:

- 2 Tilapia fillets
- 1 tbsp olive oil
- 1/2 tsp paprika
- 1/4 tsp salt
- 1/4 tsp black pepper

Optional: Squeeze of lemon juice, chopped fresh herbs

For Serving (Optional):

- Roasted vegetables (broccoli, asparagus, zucchini)
- Quinoa or brown rice pilaf
- Fresh lemon wedges and chopped parsley for garnish

Instructions

1. Firstly, pat the fish fillets dry with paper towels to remove any excess moisture. This will help in obtaining the crispy edges and a uniformly cooked fish.
2. Put olive oil, paprika (or chosen spice blend), salt, and pepper in a small bowl. Spread this mixture evenly over the Tilapia fillets on both sides. If you like, add lemon juice or chopped herbs for more flavor.
3. Preheat your oven to 400°F (205°C). For easy cleaning purposes, line a baking sheet with parchment paper. Arrange seasoned Tilapia fillets on prepared baking sheets and cook for 15 – 20 minutes or until they are done to taste and the internal temperature reaches 145°F.
4. Transfer the Easy Baked Tilapia onto plates and serve alongside selected sides. Garnish with fresh lemon wedges and chopped parsley for some freshness and color.

Nutrition per serving:

Calories: 300 Fat: 20g Carbs: 10g Protein: 35g

Simple Garlic Shrimp

Prep time: 5 minutes Cook time: 5-7 minutes Servings: 2-3

Ingredients

For the Shrimp:

- 12 oz. raw shrimp, peeled and deveined
- 1 tbsp olive oil
- 2 cloves garlic, minced
- 1/2 tsp red pepper flakes (optional)
- 1/4 tsp salt
- 1/4 tsp black pepper
- Squeeze of lemon juice (optional)
- Chopped fresh parsley or cilantro for garnish (optional)

For Serving (Optional):

- Brown rice or quinoa pilaf
- Steamed vegetables

- Fresh lemon wedges

Instructions

1. Place the shrimp on a paper towel to get rid of water. This is important for better browning and flavor uptake.
2. Place a large skillet over medium heat; add olive oil and heat. Add minced garlic and cook for 30 seconds until fragrant or its aroma is released. Add red pepper flakes if you want (if using). Cook again, then another 15 seconds.
3. Put the shrimp into the pan, flipping it over after 2-3 minutes per side or when it turns pink and white. The inside temperature should be at least 145 F to eat.
4. Season it with salt and black pepper once it is cooked. If desired, squeeze some lemon juice on top for added freshness.
5. The Simple Garlic Shrimp served with chopped cilantro or parsley as a garnish will have superb coloration and scent when placed on the plates. Consume with your preferred sides and enjoy the lively, garlicky tastiness!

Nutrition per serving:

Calories: 200 Fat: 10g Carbs: 10g Protein: 25g

Grilled Scallops

Prep time: 10 minutes Cook time: 4-6 minutes Servings: 2-3

Ingredients

For the Scallops:

- 12 large sea scallops
- 1 tbsp olive oil
- 1/2 tsp lemon zest
- 1/4 tsp paprika
- 1/4 tsp garlic powder
- 1/4 tsp salt
- 1/4 tsp black pepper

Optional: Pinch of cayenne pepper, chopped fresh herbs

For Serving (Optional):

- Grilled skewers of vegetables
- Quinoa or brown rice pilaf
- Fresh lemon wedges and chopped parsley for garnish

Instructions

1. Remove the excess moisture by gently patting the scallops using a towel. Doing so prevents them from sticking and allows them to brown evenly.
2. Whisk together olive oil, lemon zest, paprika, garlic powder, salt, and pepper in a small bowl. Adding a little/ tiny chopped herbs or a pinch of cayenne pepper is possible for those who prefer it spicier. Dip the scallops into the marinade until coated evenly.

3. Preheat your grill on medium-high heat. Lightly oil grates to prevent sticking.

4. Either skewer scallops or put them directly on the grill. When cooking, they will become golden brown and opaque within 2-3 minutes per side. Note that overcooking should be avoided as scallops tend to become tough quickly.

5. Take the Grilled Scallops onto plates while arranging your chosen sides next to them. Finally, garnish with fresh lemon wedges and chopped parsley.

Nutrition per serving:

Calories: 200 Fat: 10g Carbs: 10g Protein: 25g

Baked Whole Crappie

Prep time: 10 minutes Cook time: 15-20 minutes Servings: 4

Ingredients

For the Crappie:

- 4 whole crappie (6-8 oz each), cleaned and scaled
- 1 tbsp olive oil
- 1/2 tsp paprika or your favorite herb and spice blend
- 1/4 tsp salt
- 1/4 tsp black pepper
- Squeeze of lemon juice (optional)
- Chopped fresh herbs like parsley or dill

For Serving (Optional):

- Roasted vegetables
- Quinoa or brown rice pilaf
- Fresh lemon wedges and chopped parsley for garnish

Instructions

1. Spray the cleaned crappie gently and dry them using a paper towel. Such helps to ensure that the skin is crispy while cooking remains even.

2. Mix olive oil, paprika (or any spice of your choice), salt, and pepper in a small bowl. Apply this mix on both sides of the crappie evenly. Optionally, a squirt of lemon juice or fresh herbs can be added for extra zest.

3. Preheat your oven to 400°F. Cover a baking sheet with parchment paper for easy cleaning purposes. Put the well-seasoned crappie on the baking sheet and bake it for approximately 15-20 minutes until the internal temperature reaches 145°F, cooked through.

4. Place Baked Whole Crappie on plates and serve with selected sides. Use fresh lemon wedges and chopped parsley to garnish and brighten it.

Nutrition per serving:

Calories: 300 Fat: 15g Carbs: 10g Protein: 35g

Pan-Seared Red Snapper

Prep time: 5 minutes Cook time: 8-10 minutes Servings: 2

Ingredients:

For the Red Snapper:

- 2 Red Snapper fillets
- 1 tbsp olive oil
- 1/2 tsp paprika or your favorite herb and spice blend
- 1/4 tsp salt
- 1/4 tsp black pepper
- Squeeze of lemon juice
- Chopped fresh herbs like parsley

For Serving (Optional):

- Roasted vegetables
- Quinoa or brown rice pilaf
- Fresh lemon wedges and chopped parsley for garnish

Instructions

1. To remove excess water, Pat dry the fish fillets with paper towels. This will ensure that the skin gets crispy and evenly browned.
2. Mix olive oil, paprika (or other spices), salt and pepper in a small bowl. Apply the mixture evenly to both sides of the Red Snapper fillets. Add a squeeze of lemon juice or chopped fresh herbs for extra flavor.
3. Put a large skillet on medium heat until it gets boiling and begins to shimmer. Add the Red Snapper fillets while avoiding overcrowding.
4. On each side of the fish, cook for 3-4 minutes or until golden brown and well done. The inside temperature should reach 145°F for safe eating.
5. Put the Pan-Seared Red Snapper on a plate and rest for about 5 minutes before serving. It will help maximize flavor and tenderness by letting juices redistribute through fish.
6. Choose your favorite sides with Pan-Seared Red Snapper. Finish off with fresh wedges of lemon and chopped parsley on top.

Nutrition per serving:

Calories: 350 Fat: 20g Carbs: 10g Protein: 35g

CHAPTER 7: VEGETABLE RECIPES

Easy Roasted Broccoli

Prep time: 5 minutes Cook time: 15-20 minutes Servings: 4-6

Ingredients:

For the Broccoli:

- 1 head of broccoli, cut into florets
- 1 tbsp olive oil
- 1/2 tsp salt
- 1/4 tsp black pepper

Optional: Pinch of chili flakes, garlic powder

For Serving (Optional):

- Lemon wedges
- Parmesan cheese (optional)
- Roasted vegetables
- Quinoa or brown rice

Instructions

1. Cut off the broccoli head and slice it into small pieces as you would like to eat them. Discard the vast stalks. After that, dry the florets using paper towels to remove any additional water that will cause uneven browning.
2. In a large bowl, Olive oil, salt, and pepper blend with broccoli florets. If you want an additional punch, add chili flakes, garlic powder, or your favorite seasoning mix by sprinkling a little bit on your florets and tossing them until they are well-coated.
3. The seasoned broccoli florets are then spread out into one layer on a baking sheet lined with parchment paper. For best results, ensure proper airflow and even browning. Then preheat your oven to 425°F (220°C).
4. Roast the broccoli for 15-20 minutes until it is lightly browned and crisp-tender. Internal temperature should reach at least 145°F for safe consumption. Halfway through roasting, flip the florets so that they cook evenly.

Nutrition per serving

Calories: 100 Fat: 10g Carbs: 5g Protein: 3g

Roasted Garlic Lemon Broccoli

Prep time: 10 minutes Cook time: 15-20 minutes Servings: 4-6

Ingredients:

For the Broccoli:

- 1 head of broccoli, cut into florets
- 2 tbsp olive oil
- 1/2 tsp salt
- 1/4 tsp black pepper

- 1/4 tsp crushed red pepper flakes (optional)
- 4 whole garlic cloves, unpeeled
- Juice of 1/2 lemon

For Serving (Optional):

- Lemon wedges
- Parmesan cheese (optional)
- Grilled chicken or fish
- Quinoa or brown rice

Instructions

1. Start by washing the broccoli and divide it into small florets that are easy to chew. Remove the stems that are too thick for consumption. Remove any excess moisture by taking paper towels and patting the florets dry so they can brown evenly.
2. Put salt, olive oil, pepper, and red pepper flakes for the dressing if you like it hot. Mix well.
3. On a parchment paper resulting from a baking sheet, lay out the oiled broccoli pieces.
4. Sprinkle lemon juice over the garlic and broccoli.
5. Set the oven at 425°F (220 °C) and bake for 15-20 minutes until it is cooked but still crunchy. The cloves should be tender and slightly deep in color. Cook them halfway through by turning them over.

Nutrition per serving:

Calories: 100 Fat: 10g Carbs: 10g Protein: 4g

Broccoli Cranberry Salad

Prep time: 15 minutes Cook time: 5 minutes Servings: 4-6

Ingredients

For the Salad:

- 3 cups of broccoli florets, blanched or lightly steamed
- 1 cup of dried cranberries
- 1/2 cup of crumbled feta cheese
- 1/4 cup of chopped walnuts or pecans (toasted)
- 1/4 cup of red onion, thinly sliced
- Optional: Chopped fresh herbs like parsley or dill

For the Dressing:

- 2 tbsp olive oil
- 1 tbsp lemon juice
- 1 tsp Dijon mustard
- 1/4 tsp honey or maple syrup
- Salt and black pepper to taste

Instructions

1. Steam the florets of broccoli until they are just tender. Drain and let them cool slightly if you would like to, and chop them into small pieces.
2. Mix the parboiled broccoli florets with dried cranberries, feta cheese, toasted nuts, and red onion in a large bowl.
3. Whisk the olive oil, lemon juice, Dijon mustard, honey or maple syrup, salt, and pepper in a small bowl. Drizzle it over the salad and mix well.

4. To add a tangy twist, sprinkle chopped fresh herbs such as parsley or dill.

5. Transfer the Broccoli Cranberry Salad to a serving bowl and allow it to stand for a few minutes to blend the flavors. You can enjoy it as a light lunchtime meal, a refreshing complement to a meal, or even as a healthy snack at any time of day.

Nutrition per serving:

Calories: 250 Fat: 15g Carbs: 25g Protein: 10g

Raw Cauliflower Salad

Prep time: 15 minutes Servings: 4-6

Ingredients:

For the Salad:

- 1 medium head cauliflower, cut into florets
- 1 cup of chopped cucumber
- 1/2 cup of chopped red bell pepper
- 1/4 cup of chopped red onion (optional)
- 1/4 cup of raisins or dried cranberries
- 1/4 cup of sunflower seeds or pumpkin seeds

Optional: Chopped fresh herbs like parsley or dill

For the Dressing:

- 2 tbsp olive oil
- 1 tbsp lemon juice
- 1 tsp Dijon mustard
- 1/4 tsp honey or maple syrup
- Pinch of salt and black pepper

Instructions

1. Chop the cauliflower head into florets and grate them using a box grater or food processor. That creates a soft and tiny foundation for the salad.

2. Mix in grated cauliflower, diced cucumber, red bell pepper, purple onion (if you have any), sultanas or dried cranberries, sunflower, or pumpkin seeds.

3. Mix olive oil, lemon juice, Dijon mustard, honey or maple syrup, salt, and pepper in a small bowl while continuously whisking. Let the dressing spread over the salad when it's tossed up.

4. For an added kick of taste and aroma, garnish with finely chopped fresh herbs like parsley or dill.

Nutrition per serving:

Calories: 200 Fat: 10g Carbs: 15g Protein: 5g

Cauliflower Tabbouleh

Prep time: 15 minutes Servings: 4-6

Ingredients

For the Salad:

- 1 medium head cauliflower, grated
- 1 cup of chopped cucumber
- 1 cup of chopped cherry tomatoes
- 1/2 cup of chopped red onion
- 1/4 cup of chopped fresh parsley
- 1/4 cup of chopped fresh mint
- 1/4 cup of chopped Kalamata olives (optional)
- 1/4 cup of crumbled feta cheese (optional)

For the Dressing:

- 3 tbsp olive oil
- 2 tbsp lemon juice
- 1/2 tsp garlic powder
- 1/4 tsp salt
- Pinch of black pepper

Instructions

1. Shred the cauliflower with a box grater or in a mixer. This gives it a couscous-like texture that imitates the bulgur used in traditional tabbouleh.
2. In a big bowl, mix the grated cauliflower, chopped cucumber, cherry tomatoes, red onion, parsley, mint, Kalamata olives (if using), and crumbled feta cheese (if using).
3. Mix olive oil, lemon juice, garlic powder, salt, and pepper in another small bowl. Put dressing over salad and toss it until everything is coated well.
4. Put the top on the bowl inside a refrigerator for at least 30 minutes to lightly soften flavor mixes, and the caul soften is optional; this step improves its texture and taste.

Nutrition per serving:

Calories: 200 Fat: 10g Carbs: 10g Protein: 5g

Spicy Marinated Cauliflower Salad

Prep time: 15 minutes Servings: 4-6

Ingredients

For the Salad:

- 1 medium head cauliflower, cut into florets
- 1/2 cup of chopped cucumber
- 1/4 cup of chopped red onion
- 1/4 cup of chopped red bell pepper
- 1/4 cup of chopped fresh cilantro
- 1/4 cup of crumbled feta cheese (optional)

For the Marinade:

- 2 tbsp olive oil
- 1 tbsp lime juice
- 1 tsp sriracha or chili paste
- 1/2 tsp grated ginger
- 1/4 tsp cumin
- Pinch of salt and black pepper

Instructions

1. Divide the head of cauliflower into bite-sized florets. Blanching for 2-3 minutes will give them a less complex texture, but it's unnecessary.
2. Mix olive oil, lime juice, sriracha or chili paste, grated ginger, cumin, salt, and pepper in a small bowl. It is this which makes a fiery marinade to favorite the cauliflower.
3. Transfer the cauliflower florets into a big bowl and pour the marinade over them. Toss to even out and ensure all florets get spiced up. Cover and refrigerate for at least 30 minutes or overnight to maximize the absorption of flavors.
4. Add chopped cucumber, red bell pepper, and cauliflower to prepare. Toss gently to mix it.
5. Finally, sprinkle with chopped fresh cilantro. And if you want to make it a bit more creamy and salty, add crumbled feta cheese (optional).

Nutrition per serving:

Calories: 200 Fat: 15g Carbs: 10g
Protein: 5g

Whole Plant Chopped Salad

Prep time: 15 minutes Cook time: 10-15 minutes Servings: 4-6

Ingredients

For the Salad:

- 2 cups of mixed greens (kale, spinach, arugula)
- 1 cup of broccoli florets, roasted or blanched
- 1 cup of zucchini, chopped and roasted
- 1/2 cup of chopped red bell pepper
- 1/2 cup of chopped cucumber
- 1/4 cup of halved cherry tomatoes
- 1/4 cup of sliced red onion (optional)
- 1/4 cup of cooked quinoa or brown rice (optional)
- 1/2 avocado, sliced

For the Dressing:

- 2 tbsp olive oil
- 1 tbsp lemon juice
- 1 tsp Dijon mustard
- 1/2 tsp maple syrup or honey
- 1/4 tsp dried oregano
- Pinch of salt and black pepper

Instructions

1. Slice the greens, red bell pepper, cucumber, or red onion (optional). Boil or bake the florets in the oven until tender-crisp. The zucchini cubes should be roasted until they are slightly softened and caramelized.
2. Put the roasted broccoli, chopped red bell pepper, roasted zucchini, mixed greens, cherry tomatoes, cucumber, red onion (if using), quinoa, or brown rice (if using) into

a large bowl. Mix gently to avoid damaging the leaves.

3. In a small bowl, whisk together olive oil, lemon juice, mustard powder, maple syrup or honey, dried oregano, salt, and pepper till well blended. Pour it all over the salad and toss lightly.

4. On top of the salad, place slices of avocado; serve immediately.

Nutrition per serving

Calories: 350 Fat: 20g Carbs: 35g Protein: 15g Fiber: 10g

Whole Plant Chopped Salad

Prep time: 20 minutes Cook time: 15 minutes Servings: 4-6

Ingredients

For the Salad:

- 2 cups of mixed greens
- 1 cup of quinoa, cooked and cooled
- 1 mango, chopped
- 1/2 cup of pineapple, chopped
- 1/2 cup of jicama, chopped
- 1/4 cup of red bell pepper, chopped
- 1/4 cup of red onion, thinly sliced
- 1/4 cup of chopped fresh cilantro
- 1/4 cup of crumbled cashews

For the Dressing:

- 2 tbsp olive oil
- 1 tbsp lime juice
- 1 tsp orange juice
- 1/2 tsp honey
- 1/4 tsp chili flakes
- Pinch of salt and black pepper

Instructions

1. Chop and wash the leaves, tomato, pepper, and onion. Prepare quinoa as directed on pack and allow to cool. Peel and cut a mango, a pineapple, and a jicama.

2. Add mixed greens, cooled quinoa, chopped mango, pineapple, jicama, red bell pepper, red onion, and chopped cilantro in a large bowl. Toss lightly without tearing the salad leaves.

3. In a small cup, put together the olive oil, lime juice, orange juice, honey chili flakes, and salt pepper. Pour over the salad; mix well.

4. Scatter crumbled cashews onto the salad top immediately before serving.

Nutrition per serving:

Calories: 400 Fat: 15g Carbs: 45g Protein: 15g Fiber: 5g

Fast and Easy Creamed Spinach

Prep time: 10 minutes Cook time: 15-20 minutes Servings: 4-6

Ingredients

For the Spinach:

- 1 lb. fresh spinach, washed and roughly chopped
- 2 tbsp butter
- 1/4 cup of chopped onion
- 1/4 tsp garlic powder

For the Sauce:

- 2 tbsp milk
- 2 tbsp all-purpose flour
- 1 cup of chicken broth
- 1/4 cup of grated Parmesan cheese (optional)
- Pinch of salt and black pepper

Instructions

1. The butter should be melted in a large saucepan over medium heat. Add the onion that has been cut into pieces and cook it until soft, for about 3 minutes.
2. Put the spinach that has been washed and chopped into the pot and cook it by flipping it once in a while until it becomes soft and reduces in size. This is an excellent time to add garlic powder for a smoky flavor.
3. Pour milk with flour into a small bowl after whisking them for smoothness. The mixture should be poured over the cooked spinach while stirring until thickening. Chicken broth can then be slowly added, whisking continuously as one does so till all forms part of a smooth sauce.
4. Lastly, if you desire more of a creamy texture and rich flavor, stir in grated Parmesan cheese. Season with salt and freshly ground black pepper to taste.

Nutrition per serving:

Calories: 150 Fat: 10g Carbs: 5g Protein: 10g

Roasted Brussels Sprouts

Prep time: 10 minutes Cook time: 20-25 minutes Servings: 4-6

Ingredients

- 1 lb. Brussels sprouts, trimmed and halved
- 2 tbsp olive oil
- 1/2 tsp salt
- 1/4 tsp black pepper

Optional: Additional seasonings like garlic powder, smoked paprika, or chili flakes

Instructions

1. Preheat your oven to 400°F (200°C). Trim the edges of Brussels sprouts and slice them vertically into halves or in quarters for large sizes.
2. Toss olive oil, salt, and black pepper in a bowl of prepared

Brussels sprouts. To make it tastier, you can use other spices, such as garlic powder or chili flakes.

3. Spread seasoned Brussels sprouts out flat onto a baking sheet. Don't overcrowd the pan so they don't all brown at once. Roast until tender and crisp at the edges – 20–25 minutes.

4. Halfway through roasting, stir Brussels sprouts for even browning. Remove from oven once golden brown and tender-crisp.

Nutrition per serving:

Calories: 80 Fat: 6g Carbs: 10g Protein: 3g Fiber: 4g

Sautéed Lacinato Kale

Prep time: 5 minutes Cook time: 10 minutes Servings: 4-6

Ingredients

For the Kale:

- 1 bunch lacinato kale, ribs removed and roughly chopped
- 1 tbsp olive oil
- 2 cloves garlic, minced
- Pinch of red pepper flakes (optional)

For the Sauce:

- 1/4 cup of chicken broth
- 1 tbsp lemon juice
- Salt and black pepper to taste

Instructions

1. Wash and remove the tough stems from the lacinato kale. Roughly cut up the leaves.

2. Heat olive oil in a large frying pan over medium heat. Mix garlic and cook until it has a scent, approximately 30 seconds. For some zing, throw in some red pepper flakes.

3. Add these chopped kale and toss with garlic oil until it is coated. Sauté for about 4 minutes, stirring occasionally until the kale wilts slightly. Don't cook too much as it should remain bright green.

4. Pour in chicken broth (or vegetable broth) and lemon juice. Stir well to mix everything and season with salt and black pepper to taste. Bring to a simmer, reduce heat for 1-2min until it thickens slightly, stirring occasionally.

Nutrition per serving:

Calories: 60 Fat: 4g Carbs: 5g Protein: 2g Fiber: 3g

Quick and Easy Sautéed Spinach

Prep time: 5 minutes Cook time: 5 minutes Servings: 4-6

Ingredients

For the Spinach:

- 1 lb. fresh spinach, washed
- 1 tbsp olive oil
- 1-2 cloves garlic, minced
- Pinch of red pepper flakes (optional)

For the Sauce:

- 1/4 cup of chicken broth
- 1 tbsp lemon juice
- Salt and black pepper to taste

Instructions

1. Thoroughly wash the fresh spinach and cut off any tough stalks. You can chop the leaves roughly or leave them whole, depending on your preference.

2. In a big skillet, warm the olive oil over medium heat. Add the minced garlic and heat for 30 seconds or until fragrant. You can optionally add a sprinkle of red pepper flakes for a slight kick.

3. Toss to coat the spinach with the garlic oil after adding the cleaned spinach. Saute the spinach for two to three minutes, stirring now and again, until it wilts and shrinks significantly. It should keep its brilliant green color and delicate texture, so be careful not to overcook it.

4. Add the lemon juice and chicken or vegetable broth. After combining, taste and add more salt and black pepper if needed. Simmer the sauce for another minute or two or until it thickens slightly.

Nutrition per serving:

Calories: 60 Fat: 4g Carbs: 6g Protein: 3g Fiber: 3g

Fresh Strawberry Granita

Prep time: 10 minutes Chilling Time: 4 hours or more Servings: 4-6

Ingredients

- 1 lb. fresh strawberries, hulled and halved
- 1/2 cup of sugar
- 1 tbsp lemon juice
- 2 tbsp water

Instructions

1. Place the halved strawberries, water, lemon juice, and sugar in a blender. Blend until well integrated and smooth.
2. Pour the strawberry mixture into a shallow baking dish or pan. Freeze for four hours or longer or until slushy and partially frozen. Every 30 to 60 minutes, scrape the frozen mixture with a fork to break up the larger ice crystals and produce a fluffy, light granita texture.
3. Spoon the strawberry granita into bowls or glasses after it's frothy and fluffy. Serve immediately as an excellent dessert or a way to clear your palette.

Nutrition per serving:

Calories: 200 Fat: 0g Carbs: 50g
Protein: 1g Fiber: 2g

Chia Seed Pudding

Prep time: 5 minutes Soaking Time: 4 hours Servings: 1

Ingredients

Basic Chia Pudding:

- 2 tbsp chia seeds
- 1/2 cup of milk (dairy or plant-based)
- 1 tsp sweetener
- 1/4 tsp vanilla extract (optional)

Optional Add-Ins:

- Fresh fruit
- Chopped nuts or seeds
- Nut butter swirl
- Spices like cinnamon, nutmeg, or cardamom

Instructions

1. Place the chia seeds, milk, sweetener, and optional vanilla essence in a glass or container with a cover. Give it a good stir to make sure everything is dispersed equally.
2. Put the jar in the refrigerator for at least four hours, or better yet, overnight. As the chia seeds absorb the liquid, they thicken and take on the consistency of a pudding.
3. Be imaginative! Add as much or as little as you wish to your chia pudding: chopped nuts or seeds,

fresh fruit, nut butter swirls, or spices.

4. Scoop up some creamy chia seed pudding and enjoy it with a spoon! Savor it for breakfast, a light snack, or even dessert.

Nutrition per serving:

Calories: 250 Fat: 10g Carbs: 20g Protein: 5g Fiber: 10g

Fresh No-Bake Fruit Pie

Prep time: 15 minutes Chilling Time: 2 hours Servings: 6-8

Ingredients

For the Crust:

- 1 1/2 cups of graham cracker crumbs
- 1/2 cup of chopped nuts
- 1/4 cup of melted butter
- 2 tbsp honey or maple syrup

For the Filling:

- 2 cups of mixed fresh berries
- 1/2 cup of sliced stone fruit
- 1/4 cup of freshly squeezed lemon juice
- 2 tbsp cornstarch
- 2 tbsp honey or maple syrup
- 1/4 tsp vanilla extract

Instructions

1. Preheat oven to 350°F (175°C). Mix crushed digestive biscuits, chopped nuts, melted butter, and honey or maple syrup in a large bowl until everything comes together and the dough becomes pressable. Press evenly onto the base and sides of the 9-inch pie plate. Bake for 10 minutes and then cool on a wire rack.
2. Put mixed berries, stone fruit (if using), lemon juice, cornstarch, honey or maple syrup, and vanilla extract in a saucepan. Bring to medium heat; stir constantly until thickened and bubbles form. Turn down the heat to low; simmer gently for 5–7 minutes until the fruit softens and the filling resembles jam.
3. Pour hot fruit mixture into cooled graham crust. Cool completely at room temperature for at least 2 hours or refrigerate to firm up.
4. Cut the pie into slices and serve cold with whipped cream, fresh fruits, or a drizzle of honey if desired.

Nutrition per serving:

Calories: 300 Fat: 15g Carbs: 35g Protein: 3g Fiber: 7g

Green No-Bean Hummus

Prep time: 10 minutes Cook time: 10 minutes Servings: 4-6

Ingredients

- 2 cups of broccoli florets, blanched or steamed
- 1 ripe avocado, peeled and pitted
- 1/2 cup of fresh basil leaves
- 1/4 cup of tahini
- 2 tbsp olive oil
- 2 tbsp lemon juice
- 1/4 tsp garlic powder
- Pinch of salt and black pepper

Instructions

1. Put a combination of blanched or steamed broccoli florets, avocado, basil leaves, tahini, olive oil, lemon juice, garlic powder, salt, and black pepper in a food processor.
2. Blend until smooth and creamy while occasionally scraping down the sides. If desired, add more lemon juice or salt to taste.
3. The green hummus should then be taken to a serving bowl. For a pop of color, drizzle with extra olive oil and garnish with fresh parsley or dill. Use it with veggie sticks, pita bread, crackers, or even a salad dressing!

Nutrition per serving:

Calories: 200 Fat: 15g Carbs: 15g
Protein: 7g Fiber: 5g

Pineapple Cranberry Salad

Prep time: 10 minutes Servings: 4-6

Ingredients:

- 1 cup of chopped fresh pineapple
- 1/2 cup of fresh cranberries
- 1/2 cup of red grapes, halved
- 1/4 cup of chopped pecans
- 1/4 cup of crumbled feta cheese (optional)
- Handful of fresh mint leaves, chopped (optional)

Dressing:

- 2 tbsp olive oil
- 1 tbsp honey or maple syrup
- 1 tbsp lime juice
- 1/4 tsp ground ginger
- Pinch of salt and black pepper

Instructions

1. The diced pineapple, cranberries, grapes, and pecans should all be mixed in a big bowl.
2. Crumble the feta cheese on top of the fruit and nut combination. To add a cool touch, add chopped mint leaves.
3. Mix the olive oil, ground ginger, lime juice, honey or maple syrup, salt, and black pepper in a small bowl.
4. After drizzling the salad with the dressing, gently toss to coat. To ensure optimal freshness, serve immediately and enjoy the explosion of flavors with every bite!

Nutrition per serving:

Calories: 200 Fat: 15g Carbs: 25g Protein: 3g Fiber: 4g

Classic Cherries Jubilee

Prep time: 10 minutes Freezing Time: 4 hours or more Servings: 4-6

Ingredients:

- 1 lb. fresh blueberries
- 1/2 cup of sugar
- 1 tbsp lemon juice
- 2 tbsp water

Instructions

1. Mix blueberries, sugar, lemon juice, and water in a blender. Blend until the mixture is smooth and consistent.
2. Put the blueberry mixture into a shallow baking dish or pan. Freeze for about four hours or until it begins to solidify but remains slushy. Remember to scrape it with a fork every half an hour to one hour so that you can create smaller ice crystals, hence fluffy granita.
3. When it is frozen and fluffy, scoop it into bowls or glasses. It is perfect when served as soon as possible after making it a refreshing dessert or palate cleanser.
4. Sieve the blended blueberry mixture before freezing.
5. You can also add a little blueberry syrup or liqueur if you like.

6. Before adding the simple syrup to the mixture of blueberries, infuse it with basil or mint leaves.
7. You can also top your shaved ice with some chilled sparkling water or prosecco for a fizzy surprise if you so wish.

Nutrition per serving:

Calories: 200 Fat: 0g Carbs: 50g Protein: 1g Fiber: 2g

Ground Cherry Pie

Prep time: 30 minutes Cook time: 50-60 minutes Servings: 6-8

Ingredients

For the Crust:

- 1 1/2 cups of all-purpose flour
- 1/2 tsp salt
- 1/2 cup of cold unsalted butter, cubed
- 3-4 tbsp ice water

For the Filling:

- 2 lb. fresh ground cherries, husked
- 1/2 cup of sugar
- 1/4 cup of cornstarch
- 1/4 tsp ground cinnamon
- Pinch of nutmeg
- 1 tbsp lemon juice
- 1 tbsp butter, softened (optional)

For the Topping:

- 1 egg yolk, beaten with 1 tbsp heavy cream

- Granulated sugar for sprinkling

Instructions

1. Mix the flour and salt in a big bowl. Work in the cubed butter with your fingertips or a pastry cutter until it resembles coarse crumbs. One tbsp at a time, drizzle in the ice water and stir until the dough comes together. The dough should be shaped into a disk, covered with plastic wrap, and chilled for at least half an hour.
2. Husky the ground cherries and wash them. Put them in a big basin with lemon juice, sugar, cornstarch, cinnamon, and nutmeg. To coat, gently toss.
3. Turn the oven on to 375°F, or 190°C. Roll out the cold dough into a 12-inch circle on a surface dusted with flour. Press the dough into the bottom and edges of a 9-inch pie dish.
4. Fill the prepared pie crust with the ground cherry mixture. If desired, add a dollop of softened butter for extra richness.
5. For a golden gloss, dust the pie crust edges with granulated sugar after brushing them with the beaten egg yolk mixture.
6. Bake the pie for fifty to sixty minutes or until the filling bubbles and the crust is golden brown. Before serving, allow to cool slightly on a wire rack.
7. Enjoy warm or room temperature, with the optional topping of whipped cream or a dollop of vanilla ice cream.

Nutrition per serving:

Calories: 400 Fat: 20g Carbs: 50g Protein: 4g Fiber: 4g

Cherry Squares

Prep time: 30 minutes Cook time: 45-50 minutes Servings: 9-12

Ingredients

For the Crust:

- 1 1/2 cups of all-purpose flour
- 1/2 tsp salt
- 1/2 cup of cold unsalted butter, cubed
- 3-4 tbsp ice water

For the Filling:

- 2 cups of fresh or frozen pitted cherries
- 1/2 cup of sugar
- 1/4 cup of cornstarch
- 1/4 tsp almond extract (optional)
- 1 tbsp lemon juice

For the Topping:

- 1/2 cup of all-purpose flour
- 1/4 cup of rolled oats
- 1/4 cup of brown sugar
- 1/4 cup of cold unsalted butter, cubed
- Pinch of cinnamon

Instructions

1. Preheat the oven to a temperature of 375°F (190°C). In a large bowl, mix flour and salt. Mix cubed butter using your fingers or pastry cutter to get loose crumbs. Drop ice water into the mixture one tbsp at a time, stirring gently until dough forms. Shape it into a disc, wrap it in plastic, and refrigerate for 30 minutes.
2. Meanwhile, cook cherries, sugar, cornstarch, almond extract (optional), and lemon juice in a saucepan until thick and bubbly. Let cool slightly.
3. Roll out the chilled dough on a lightly floured surface to form a 12-inch circle. Fit it evenly into the bottom and sides of a 9-inch square baking pan. Poke a few fork holes on the bottom so the crust does not puff up too much.
4. Pour cooled cherry filling over the prepared crust.
5. Mix flour, oats, brown sugar, butter, and cinnamon in a small bowl using your fingers or a pastry cutter until the mixture resembles coarse crumbs. Sprinkle topping evenly over cherry filling.
6. Bake cherry squares for 45-50 minutes or until the crust is golden brown and the topping is crisp and bubbly. Allow to cool slightly on a wire rack before serving.
7. Enjoy warm or at room temperature with a scoop of vanilla ice cream on top of each serving for an extra decadent treat.

Nutrition per serving:

Calories: 350 Fat: 20g Carbs: 45g Protein: 3g Fiber: 3g

Cran-Raspberry Jellies

Prep time: 15 minutes Cook time: 5 minutes Servings: 6

Ingredients

For the Jelly Base:

- 1 envelope of unflavored gelatin powder (28g)
- 1/2 cup of cold water
- 1 cup of boiling water
- 1 cup of cranberry juice
- 1/2 cup of granulated sugar

For the Raspberry Swirl:

- 1 cup of fresh raspberries, mashed
- 1 tbsp honey or maple syrup (optional)
- 1 tbsp lemon juice

Instructions

1. In a bowl, sprinkle the gelatin powder over the cold water and let it soak for 5 minutes.
2. Simmer the boiling water in a saucepan, and then remove from heat before stirring in the dissolved gelatin.
3. Put this cranberry juice and sugar into the saucepan and dissolve these sugars by stirring them.
4. Distribute the cranberry mixture evenly into six small ramekins or

molds. Chill for at least 2 hours until set.

5. Once set, purée raspberries with honey or maple syrup (if used) and lemon juice. If you want it to contrast the rest of the dish, leave some pieces larger.

6. When it is firm, gently spoon it over the raspberry mixture, creating a swirl throughout the cranberry layer. Use a toothpick or the back of a spoon to create a marbled effect if needed.

7. Let stand in refrigerator 2-3 hours longer inside until jelly has become firm and raspberry swirl is done.

8. Remove Cran-Raspberry Jellies from their molds onto small plates. Serve chilled as refreshing desserts or light elegant treats.

Nutrition per serving:

Calories: 125 Fat: 0g Carbs: 25g
Protein: 1g Fiber: 2g

Black Raspberry Cobbler

Prep time: 15 minutes Cook time: 45-50 minutes Servings: 6-8

Ingredients:

For the Filling:

- 2 cups of fresh black raspberries
- 1/2 cup of granulated sugar
- 1/4 cup of cornstarch
- 1 tbsp lemon juice
- 1 tbsp water

For the Biscuit Topping:

- 2 cups of all-purpose flour
- 2 tsp baking powder
- 1/2 tsp salt
- 1/2 cup of cold unsalted butter, cubed
- 1/2 cup of buttermilk
- 1/4 cup of granulated sugar

Instructions

1. Turn the oven on to 375°F, or 190°C. The black raspberries, sugar, cornstarch, lemon juice, and water should all be mixed in a big basin. Make sure the cornstarch is distributed evenly as you gently toss to coat.

2. Mix the flour, baking powder, and salt in another basin. Using a pastry cutter or your fingertips, cut in the cold butter until the mixture has the consistency of coarse crumbs.

3. Once the dough comes together, stir in the sugar and buttermilk (or milk combination). Avoid overmixing!

4. Fill a 9 x 13-inch baking dish with the berry mixture. Leaving some space for the berries to ooze through, place dollops of biscuit dough over the berries.

5. Bake the cobbler for 45 to 50 minutes or until the mixture bubbles and the biscuit topping is golden brown. If the filling is still a little loose, that's okay; it will solidify as it cools.

6. Before serving, allow the cobbler to cool somewhat. Savor it warm or at room temperature, and for an extra

comfortable touch, top it with whipped cream, vanilla ice cream, or honey.

Nutrition per serving:

Calories: 400 Fat: 20g Carbs: 50g Protein: 4g Fiber: 4g

Triple Berry Crisp

Prep time: 15 minutes Cook time: 40-45 minutes Servings: 6-8

Ingredients

For the Berry Filling:

- 2 cups of mixed fresh berries
- 1/4 cup of granulated sugar
- 1 tbsp cornstarch
- 1 tbsp lemon juice
- Pinch of ground cinnamon (optional)

For the Oat Topping:

- 1 cup of rolled oats
- 1/2 cup of all-purpose flour
- 1/4 cup of brown sugar
- 1/4 cup of chopped walnuts or pecans
- 1/4 cup of cold unsalted butter, cubed
- Pinch of salt

Instructions

1. Preheat the stove to 375°F (190°C). Mix the mixed berries, sugar, cornstarch, lemon juice, and cinnamon (optional). Toss it gently.

2. Mix the rolled oats, flour, brown sugar, nuts, salt, and cubed butter with your fingers or a pastry cutter until the mixture looks like crumbs that are not fine.

3. Pour the berry mixture into a 9x13-inch baking dish. Sprinkle oat topping uniformly over all berries, covering most of the fruits.

4. Bake the crisp for about forty to forty-five minutes or until its top becomes golden and the filling starts bubbling. Cool slightly before serving.

5. Eat it warm or at room temperature with a scoop of vanilla ice cream on top and whipped cream, or if you want a more exotic, sweet taste, add honey.

Nutrition per serving:

Calories: 300 Fat: 15g Carbs: 40g Protein: 4g Fiber: 3g

Grandma's Raspberry Bars

Prep time: 20 minutes Cook time: 40-45 minutes Servings: 12-15

Ingredients

For the Crust:

- 1 1/2 cups of all-purpose flour
- 1/2 tsp salt
- 1/2 cup of cold unsalted butter, cubed
- 1/4 cup of powdered sugar
- 1 large egg yolk
- 1 tbsp vanilla extract

For the Filling:

- 2 cups of fresh raspberries
- 1/2 cup of granulated sugar
- 2 tbsp cornstarch
- 1 tbsp lemon juice

For the Streusel Topping:

- 1/2 cup of all-purpose flour
- 1/4 cup of brown sugar
- 1/4 cup of chopped walnuts or pecans
- 1/4 cup of cold unsalted butter, cubed

Instructions

1. Preheat the oven to 375°F (190°C). In a large bowl, whisk together flour and salt. Blend in the cubed margarine with your fingers or pastry cutter until the texture is like coarse crumbs. Stir in powdered sugar, egg yolk, and vanilla extract until a dough ball forms. Spread dough evenly over the bottom of the ungreased 9×13-inch baking dish.
2. Mix raspberries, sugar, cornstarch, and lemon juice in another bowl. Carefully stir so that all berries will be well covered. Pour the mixture of berries over the crust prepared for it.
3. Mix brown sugar, flour, nuts, and cubed margarine in a small bowl until the mixture resembles coarse crumbs using your fingers or a pastry cutter. Sprinkle streusel topping over berries.
4. Bake raspberry bars for 40 to 45 minutes or until the crust is golden brown and the filling is bubbly. Let cool slightly; cut into bars.
5. Enjoy warm with a scoop of vanilla ice cream or whipped cream, or drizzle honey for an extra touch of indulgence at room temperature. It is also worth noting that these bars can be eaten cold as a refreshing summer snack!

Nutrition per serving:

Calories: 350 Fat: 20g Carbs: 45g
Protein: 2g Fiber: 3g